Official Journal of the European Stroke Council (ESC)
Official Journal of the European Stroke Initiative (EUSI)

Cerebrovascular Diseases

KARGER

Printed in Switzerland
on acid-free paper by
Reinhardt Druck, Basel

Appears 6-weekly:
2 volumes per year
(8 issues)

Guidelines for Authors

Cerebrovascular Diseases

Submission

Only original papers written in English are considered and should be sent to:

J. Bogousslavsky, MD
Service de Neurologie
CHUV
CH–1011 Lausanne (Switzerland)
E-Mail Julien.Bogousslavsky@chuv.hospvd.ch

or:

M.G. Hennerici, MD
Neurologische Klinik
Klinikum Mannheim der
Universität zu Heidelberg
Theodor-Kutzer-Ufer
D–68135 Mannheim (Germany)
E-Mail Hennerici@neuro.ma.uni-heidelberg.de

Manuscripts should be submitted in quadruplicate (with four sets of illustrations of which one is an original; final high-resolution pictures need only be sent after acceptance of the paper) together with a soft copy on disc. **The manuscript should match the electronic file exactly.** For details please refer to: www.karger.com/electronic_submission. Editorial work and copy-editing will be executed from the electronic version of your manuscript.

At the time of the initial submission, the paper should be accompanied by the following declaration: 'The work reported in the attached paper entitled [...] has not been and is not intended to be published anywhere except in Cerebrovascular Diseases.' The declaration should be signed by all authors.

Conditions

All manuscripts are subject to editorial review. Manuscripts are received with the explicit understanding that they are not under simultaneous consideration by any other publication. Submission of an article for publication implies transfer of the copyright from the author to the publisher upon acceptance. Accepted papers become the permanent property of 'Cerebrovascular Diseases' and may not be reproduced by any means, in whole or in part, without the written consent of the publisher. It is the author's responsibility to obtain permission to reproduce illustrations, tables, etc. from other publications.

Arrangement

Title page: The first page of each paper should indicate the title, the authors' names, the institute where the work was conducted, and a short title for use as running head.

NB: Authors wishing to preserve the phonetic meaning of diacritics (PubMed reduces diacritics to their root characters) must spell their names accordingly when submitting manuscripts (e.g. Müller should be Mueller).

Full address: The exact postal address of the corresponding author complete with postal code must be given at the bottom of the title page. Please also supply phone and fax numbers, as well as e-mail address.

Key words: For indexing purposes, a list of 3–10 key words in English is essential.

Abstract: Each paper needs an abstract of up to 10 lines. This should include the following information: *Background:* the problem that prompted the study and the purpose of the study; *Methods:* data sources, subjects, design, measurements, data analysis; *Results:* most important findings; *Conclusions:* implications, future directions.

Footnotes: Avoid footnotes.

Tables and illustrations: Tables and illustrations (both numbered in Arabic numerals) should be prepared on separate pages. Tables require a heading and figures a legend, also prepared on a separate page. For the reproduction of illustrations, only good drawings and original photographs can be accepted; negatives or photocopies cannot be used. Due to technical reasons, figures with a screen background should not be submitted. When possible, group several illustrations in one block for reproduction (max. size 180 × 223 mm) or provide crop marks. On the back of each illustration, indicate its number, the author's name, and 'top' with a soft pencil. Electronically submitted b/w halftone and color illustrations must have a final resolution of 300 dpi after scaling, line drawings one of 800–1,200 dpi.

Color illustrations: Up to 6 color illustrations per page can be integrated within the text at the special price of CHF 660.–/USD 545.00 per page. Color illustrations are reproduced at the author's expense.

References: In the text identify references by Arabic numerals [in square brackets]. Material submitted for publication but not yet accepted should be noted as 'unpublished data' and not be included in the reference list. The list of references should include only those publications which are cited in the text. Do not alphabetize; number references in the order in which they are first mentioned in the text. The surnames of the authors followed by initials should be given. There should be no punctuation other than a comma to separate the authors. Preferably, please cite all authors. Abbreviate journal names according to the Index Medicus system. (Also see International Committee of Medical Journal Editors: Uniform requirements for manuscripts submitted to biomedical journals. N Engl J Med 1997;336:309–315. www.icmje.org)

Digital Object Identifier (DOI)
S. Karger Publishers supports DOIs as unique identifiers for articles. A DOI number will be printed on the title page of each article. DOIs can be useful in the future for identifying and citing articles published online without volume or issue information. More information can be found at www.doi.org.

Examples
(a) Papers published in periodicals: Chatel J-M, Bernard H, Orson FM: Isolation and characterization of two complete Ara h 2 isoforms cDNA. Int Arch Allergy Immunol 2003;131:14–18.
(b) Papers published only with DOI numbers: Theoharides TC, Boucher W, Spear K: Serum interleukin-6 reflects disease severity and osteoporosis in mastocytosis patients. Int Arch Allergy Immunol DOI: 10.1159/000063858.
(c) Monographs: Hennerici M, Sitzer G, Weger H-D: Carotid Artery Plaques: Pathogenesis – Development – Evaluation – Treatment. Basel, Karger, 1988.
(d) Edited books: DuBois RN: Cyclooxygenase-2 and colorectal cancer; in Dannenberg AJ, Dubois RN (eds): COX-2. Prog Exp Tum Res. Basel, Karger, 2003, vol 37, pp 124–137.

Page Charges

There are no page charges for papers of 5 or fewer printed pages (including tables, illustrations and references). Each additional complete or partial page is charged to the author at CHF 275.–/USD 196.00. The allotted size of a paper is equal to approx. 13 manuscript pages (including tables, illustrations and references).

Proofs

Unless indicated otherwise, proofs are sent to the first-named author and should be returned with the least possible delay. Alterations made in proofs, other than the correction of printer's errors, are charged to the author.

Reprints

Order forms and a price list for reprints are sent with the proofs. Orders submitted after the issue is printed are subject to considerably higher prices.

KARGER

Fax +41 61 306 12 34
E-Mail karger@karger.ch
www.karger.com

The Guidelines for Authors are available at:
www.karger.com/ced_Guidelines

Cerebrovascular Diseases

General Information

Publication data: 'Cerebrovascular Diseases' is published 8 times a year. Volumes 17–18, each with 4 issues, appear in 2004.

Subscription rates: Subscriptions run for a full calendar year. Prices are given per year.

Personal subscription:

Print or Online	Print/Online combined
CHF 646.10	CHF 728.10
EUR 478.80	EUR 538.80
USD 516.60	USD 582.60

postage and handling (added to print and print/online)
CHF 42.40 Europe, CHF 62.80 Overseas
EUR 30.40
USD 42.40

Institutional subscription:

Print or Online	Print/Online combined
CHF 1846.–	CHF 1994.–
EUR 1368.–	EUR 1478.–
USD 1476.00	USD 1596.00

postage and handling (added to print and print/online)
CHF 52.80 Europe, CHF 78.40 Overseas
EUR 38.–
USD 52.80

Airmail surcharge: CHF 52.80 / USD 44.00
Subscription included in membership fee for members of the European Stroke Council (ESC)

Microforms: Please direct all enquiries and orders to:
University Microfilms Inc.
300 North Zeeb Road, P.O. Box 1346
Ann Arbor, MI 48106-1346 (USA)

Subscription orders: Orders can be placed at agencies, bookstores, directly with the Publisher
S. Karger AG, P.O. Box
CH–4009 Basel (Switzerland)
or with any of the following distributors:
Deutschland: S. Karger GmbH, Postfach
D–79095 Freiburg
France: Librairie Luginbühl
36, bd de Latour-Maubourg
F–75007 Paris
Great Britain, Ireland: S. Karger AG
4 Rickett Street
London SW6 1RU, UK
USA: S. Karger Publishers, Inc.
26 West Avon Road, P.O. Box 529
Farmington, CT 06085, USA
India, Bangladesh, Sri Lanka:
Panther Publishers Private Ltd.
33, First Main
Koramangala First Block
Bangalore 560 034, India
Japan: Karger Japan, Inc.
Yushima S Bld. 3F
4-2-3, Yushima, Bunkyo-ku
Tokyo 113-0034, Japan

Change of address: Both old and new address should be sent to the subscription source.

Single issues and back volumes: Information can be obtained through the Publisher.

Advertising: Correspondence and rate requests should be addressed to the Publisher.

Bibliographic indices: This journal is regularly listed in bibliographic services, including *Current Contents®* and Index Medicus/MEDLINE.

Copying: This journal has been registered with the Copyright Clearance Center (CCC), as indicated by the code appearing on the first page of each article. For readers in the US, this code signals consent for copying of articles for personal or internal use, or for the personal or internal use of specific clients, provided that the stated fee is paid per copy directly to
Copyright Clearance Center Inc.
222 Rosewood Drive
Danvers, MA 01923 (USA)
A copy of the first page of the article must accompany payment. Consent does not extend to copying for general distribution, for promotion, for creating new works, or for resale. In these cases, specific written permission must be obtained from the copyright owner,
S. Karger AG,
P.O. Box, CH–4009 Basel (Switzerland).

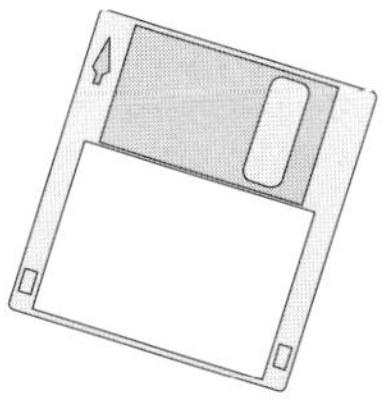

Disk Submission

A **comprehensive version** of these guidelines for the **submission of manuscripts and illustrations on disk** can be accessed online under **www.karger.com/disksubmission** or requested as a leaflet from the editorial department.

Please follow the general rules on style and arrangement in the **'Guidelines for Authors'** of the journal. Submit a **double-spaced printout** of your manuscript matching the file on disk exactly.

Technical Information

Store only data pertinent to this manuscript. Include your fonts (screen and printer fonts for Macintosh). For a **text only** manuscript, use a 3.5-inch disk. For **text and illustrations,** use 3.5 or 5.25 Magneto Optical Disc; CD-ROM (DOS or hybrid); iomega Zip/DOS (100 MB), or 44 MB, 88 MB or 200 MB SyQuest. Compress extensive data using ZIP format.

Data Description

Label your disk with the **title of the journal or book** for which it is submitted; a **short version** of the paper's title; your **name,** postal and e-mail address, fax and phone number; **hard- and software** used, including the version; and the **complete list of the file names.** File names consist of eight characters before the dot identifying the file and three characters after the dot identifying the application.

Text and Format

The **preferred word-processing package is MS-Word.** Other commonly used PC text programs and ASCII formats are accepted.
Update your data when you revise subsequent to the reviewer's or editor's decision and mark revisions clearly. Manuscripts accepted for publication are subject to **copy editing:** changes and/or questions will be marked in the manuscript, which will be returned to you with your disk and the galley proofs for checking.
Enter your text continuously flush left. Do not use any layout functions. Do not split words at the end of a line. **Do not use indentations.** Use a blank line before and a hard return at the end of paragraphs.
Arrange headings flush left. Insert only **one space after punctuation marks.** Insert Greek letters, mathematical symbols etc. with your word-processing program. Use **boldface and italics** as well as sub- and superscript where appropriate.
Tables are part of the text and should be placed at the end of the text file. Separate the individual parts of a table by lines. Use the tabulator instead of spaces. Format operation data on one line in the same column.

Legends to illustrations are part of the text and should also be listed at the end of the text file.

Illustrations

Store illustrations as separate files: do not integrate them in your text. Export **line drawings/vector graphics** as TIF, EPS or WMF format. Use Photoshop for processing and retouching **scanned half-tone images.** Save the original scan and the processed version. Export **black and white or color images** as TIF or EPS format in their anticipated size in print. **For detailed information** on how to submit illustration data on disk please consult the leaflet or **www.karger.com/disksubmission.**

KI 02 DISK

KARGER

Fax +41 61 306 12 34
E-Mail karger@karger.ch
www.karger.com

The Journal Home Page is available at:
www.karger.com/ced

European Stroke Council

Objectives

The European Stroke Council is dedicated to furthering knowledge and for promoting the prevention and treatment of stroke and cerebrovascular disorders. In addition, the Council encourages the international exchange of information, mainly within Europe. More detailed information about the European Stroke Council and its executive committee is contained in the Council's statutes, a copy of which can be obtained from the Council Secretariat.

Membership

The members of the Council are composed of neurologists, internists, surgeons, radiologists and other specialists involved in cerebrovascular research. Any recognized researcher who meets the requirements listed below is eligible to become either an active academic member, clinical member or corresponding member. Active academic members may participate in the business sessions of the Council, may vote, and are eligible for office in the Executive Committee. Clinical and corresponding members may participate in the business sessions but may not vote and are not eligible for election to office.

Active academic membership

A researcher working in Europe who:

1) has a record of research in stroke and cerebrovascular disease and also a reasonable prospect of continued activity in this research area (please attach a curriculum vitae to this application form)
2) has authored at least 2 publications dealing with stroke or cerebrovascular disease (excluding abstracts and letters) which have appeared in peer-reviewed journals with an international board in the two years preceding the application date. The applicant must be first author of at least one of the publications and co-author of a second.
3) can provide a detailed letter of support by 2 recognized investigators in the field

Clinical membership

Applies to clinicians involved in cerebrovascular disease who do not have a research record or are not involved in academic activities.

Corresponding membership

Applies to researchers working outside of Europe who meet the same requirements as those which apply to active academic membership.

Activities

The Council supports the European Stroke Conference at which the annual meetings take place. In the future, the Council aims to make provisions for bursaries and grants and intends to organize consensus meetings, encourage the development of task forces, and stimulate clinical and experimental trials.

Cerebrovascular Diseases is the official journal of the Council. A reduced-cost subscription is included in the annual membership fee.

Annual Membership Fees

Academic, clinical and corresponding members: CHF 298.–
(includes the annual subscription to *Cerebrovascular Diseases*)

If you would like to apply for membership to the European Stroke Council and fulfil the requirements listed above, please complete the application form on the reverse.

KP 01123

European Stroke Council

Application for Membership

I would like to enter an application for membership to the European Stroke Council as

- ☐ an active academic member
- ☐ a clinical member
- ☐ a corresponding member

Enclosed is a) a curriculum vitae
b) a letter of support from 2 recognized investigators in the field

Please note that applicants who meet the requirements of active academic members, but who work outside Europe will be accepted as corresponding members.

Name: ______________________________

Home Address: ______________________________

____

____

Office Address: ______________________________

____

____

Phone No.: ______________ *Fax No:* ______________

Current activities/position in research, teaching or clinical practice: ______________________________

____

____

____

Membership in other scientific societies related to stroke: ______________________________

Membership Fees

You will receive an invoice for CHF 220.– upon acceptance of your application. Membership becomes effective only after payment has been received. Do not send money now.

Please send this application together with the required C.V. and, if applicable, the letters of support, to the European Stroke Council Secretariat:

Dr. N.G. Wahlgren
Department of Neurology
Karolinska Sjukhuset
Box 60500
S–104 01 Stockholm (Sweden)

Date: ______________ Signature: ______________

Cerebrovascular
Diseases

Recommendations for Stroke Management: Update 2003

European Stroke Initiative (EUSI)

on behalf of the
European Stroke Council (ESC)
European Neurological Society (ENS)
European Federation of Neurological Societies (EFNS)

11 tables, 2004

KARGER

Basel · Freiburg · Paris · London · New York ·
Bangalore · Bangkok · Singapore · Tokyo · Sydney

Corporate Members:
Boehringer-Ingelheim
Sanofi-Synthelabo
Servier

For the European Stroke Initiative Executive Committee:
Markku Kaste, Helsinki, Finland
Werner Hacke, Heidelberg, Germany
Julien Bogousslavsky, Lausanne, Switzerland
Michael Brainin, Maria Gugging, Austria
Angel Chamorro, Barcelona, Spain
Kennedy Lees, Glasgow, United Kingdom
Didier Leys, Lille, France
Hubert Kwiecinski, Warsaw, Poland
Danilo Toni, Rome, Italy

For the EUSI Writing Committee:
Tom Skyhøj Olsen, Copenhagen, Denmark
Peter Langhorne, Glasgow, United Kingdom
Hans-Christoph Diener, Essen, Germany
Michael G. Hennerici, Mannheim, Germany
José Ferro, Lisbon, Portugal
Johani Sivenius, Kuopiu, Finland
Nils Gunnar Wahlgren, Stockholm, Sweden
Philip Bath, Nottingham, United Kingdom

Corresponding Author:
Werner Hacke, MD, PhD
Department of Neurology
University of Heidelberg
INF 400
DE–69120 Heidelberg (Germany)

S. Karger
Medical and Scientific Publishers
Basel · Freiburg · Paris · London
New York · Bangalore · Bangkok
Singapore · Tokyo · Sydney

Drug Dosage
The authors and the publisher have exerted every effort to ensure that drug selection and dosage set forth in this text are in accord with current recommendations and practice at the time of publication. However, in view of ongoing research, changes in government regulations, and the constant flow of information relating to drug therapy and drug reactions, the reader is urged to check the package insert for each drug for any change in indications and dosage and for added warnings and precautions. This is particularly important when the recommended agent is a new and/or infrequently employed drug.

Printed in Switzerland on acid-free paper by
Reinhardt Druck, Basel
ISBN 3–8055–7689–7

KARGER

Fax + 41 61 306 12 34
E-Mail karger@karger.ch
www.karger.com

Vol. 17, Suppl. 2, 2004

Cerebrovascular Diseases

Contents

KARGER

Fax + 41 61 306 12 34
E-Mail karger@karger.ch
www.karger.com

Access to full text and tables of contents, including tentative ones for forthcoming issues:
www.karger.com/ced_issues

Part 1

Cerebrovascular Diseases

Cerebrovasc Dis 2004;17(suppl 2):1–14
DOI: 10.1159/000074816

Organization of Stroke Care: Education, Referral, Emergency Management and Imaging, Stroke Units and Rehabilitation

Michael Brainin Tom Skyhøj Olsen Angel Chamorro
Hans-Christoph Diener José Ferro Michael G. Hennerici Peter Langhorne
Johani Sivenius
for the EUSI Executive Committee and the EUSI Writing Committee

Introduction

Acute stroke is one of the leading factors of morbidity and mortality worldwide. After cardiovascular disease, stroke ranks as either second or third most common cause of death in industrialized countries. In Europe, the crude death rate ranges from 63.5/100,000 (males, Switzerland, 1992) to 273.4/100,000 (females, Russia, 1991). Such large differences in mortality between east and west in Europe have been noted [Stegmayr et al., 2000] and attributed to differences in risk factor expressions, with higher levels of hypertension and other risks in eastern countries as compared with the west, thus resulting in more severe strokes in Eastern Europe [Ryglewicz et al., 2000; Brainin et al., 2000]. Within Europe, notable regional variations of stroke severity [Wolfe et al., 2000] and stroke treatment [Thomassen et al., 2003] have been reported. Stroke as the most important cause of morbidity and long-term disability in Europe imposes an enormous economic burden. The average cost from first stroke to death has been calculated for several European countries [Kaste et al., 1998] and has for example in Sweden been shown to amount to approximately 79,000 EUR [Asplund et al., 1993].

Over the past decade, acute stroke has increasingly been recognized as a medical emergency. Acute, postacute, and rehabilitation care of stroke patients in specialized wards as well as revascularizing therapies have been proven to be effective in acute ischaemic stroke. The establishment of a network consisting of acute stroke units, seamless continuation to postacute care and rehabilitation, as well as further care in the community has become standard treatment in many European countries. Systems of care have emerged that include nationwide concepts of stroke care units focusing on the acute care such as in Austria or Germany [Weimar et al., 2002; Brainin and Steiner 2003], and systems of stroke units focusing on comprehensive care including rehabilitation as in the UK or Scandinavia [Jørgensen et al., 1995; Kalra and Eade, 1995; Indredavik et al., 1997].

Considering the available scientific evidence favouring the set-up of stroke care in specialized units, several European guidelines and consensus papers have been published over the past years. These include reports from the Pan European Consensus Meeting on Stroke Management [Aboderin et al., 1996], the European Ad Hoc Consensus Group [The European Ad Hoc Consensus Group, 1996, 1997], the Task Force on Acute Neurological Stroke Care of the European Federation of Neurological Societies [Brainin et al., 1997, 2000; Thomassen et al., 2003], and the European Stroke Initiative (EUSI) [European Stroke Initiative, 2000]. North American guidelines and treatment recommendations issued by the American Academy of Neurology include those for acute treatment [Adams et al., 1994], carotid surgery [Biller et al., 1998], management of transient ischaemic attacks [Feinberg et

KARGER
Fax + 41 61 306 12 34
E-Mail karger@karger.ch
www.karger.com

1015–9770/04/0176–0001$21.00/0

Accessible online at:
www.karger.com/ced

Table 1. Definitions of levels of evidence and classes of recommendations used in this article

Level I	Highest level of evidence
Sources	1 Primary end point from randomized, double-blinded study with adequate sample size 2 Properly performed meta-analysis of qualitatively outstanding randomized trials
Level II	Intermediate level of evidence
Sources	1 Randomized, non-blinded studies 2 Small, randomized trials 3 Pre-defined secondary end points of large, randomized trials
Level III	Lower level of evidence
Sources	1 Prospective case series with concurrent or historical control 2 Post hoc analyses of randomized trials
Level IV	Undetermined level of evidence
Sources	1 Small case series without control, case reports 2 General agreement despite lack of evidence from controlled trials

al., 1994] and primary prevention of stroke [Goldstein et al., 2001]. Earlier recommendations have been issued by the WHO [WHO Task Force on Stroke and Other Cerebrovascular Disorders, 1989].

The recommendations from the EUSI published in 2000 [European Stroke Initiative, 2000] have now been completely revised and updated. In accordance with the European Neurological Society, the European Federation of Neurological Society and the European Stroke Council, which also represents the European Stroke Conference, they provide an overview of established or widely used therapeutic strategies as well as an evaluation of involving, but not yet proven strategies. These are discussed in detail as well as classified according to their scientific levels of evidence. On the basis of such evidence, specific recommendations are made. (Experts' opinions on several issues of stroke prevention and treatment can be assessed at the EUSI website 'Virtual Stroke University' free of charge at www.eusi-stroke.com. These lectures represent an extension of many issues discussed in these recommendations, but have not passed the consensus process of the EUSI documents and therefore only reflect the opinion of the lecturing expert).

The levels of evidence in this article remain unchanged as in the previous recommendations. They correspond to those published by the European Federation of Neurological Society [Hughes et al., 2001] and are listed in table 1.

Education

Public Education

Many patients and relatives do not recognize the symptoms of stroke and do not realize that seeking treatment is urgent. Reasons for this shortcoming include a poor awareness of stroke by the victim or family, reluctance to seek immediate medical help, incorrect diagnosis by the paramedical service and rating stroke as a non-emergency by medical personnel and the family physician [Becker et al., 2001; Yoon and Byles 2002; Evenson et al., 2001]. These facts emphasize the need for an ongoing education programme. The benefits of media campaigns to raise awareness of stroke have been documented in a number of studies [Becker et al., 2001; The European Ad Hoc Consensus Group, 1996]. Education programmes can be extensive and involve radio and television interviews, newspaper articles, lectures to local and regional primary care and emergency department physicians, and mailings to local physicians. The aims of public education initiatives are to enable and encourage the general population to immediately recognize the symptoms of stroke, to realize that urgent medical attention is needed and to use the emergency transportation services and immediately go to the correct hospital. Primary contact with general practitioners (GPs) may cause delays and prevent an early start of adequate therapy [Evenson et al., 2001]. Educational efforts should be directed to patients at risk for stroke, their families, caregivers or co-workers and to large employers [Wein et al., 2000]. Teaching the public about symptoms and signs of stroke is one of the highest priorities of public medical education.

Professional Education

Professional groups who must be motivated in stroke care include emergency medicine physicians and technicians, other specialists, nurses, GPs and paramedical personnel. In many European countries, neurologists have become interested in the care of stroke patients and made themselves available for this task. Stroke units are frequently part of neurology departments. However, internists, geriatricians, GPs and emergency medicine physicians may also be responsible for treating stroke patients. Due to the low number of neurologists or other stroke physicians in some European countries, many stroke patients are still not seen by a physician with special expertise in stroke management. Primary care physicians are not so much involved in the recognition of stroke as they are often bypassed via the emergency medical services (EMS) system. Therefore, they are not primarily responsible for speeding up the admission times to emergency stroke care. However, they still represent a target group for education campaigns, as they will be responsible for continuing the secondary prevention after the acute phase.

Inaccurate initial diagnosis represents a major problem. Ambulance dispatchers may have a false-positive assessment rate of up to 50%, and even in trained paramedics, this rate is about 25% [Kothari et al., 1997]. However, this result can be improved by adequate training [Kothari et al., 1997].

Paramedics and physicians also need to be trained in the recognition of symptoms and signs of acute stroke and the necessity of immediate transportation to an adequately equipped unit. The medical personnel should be trained in recognizing the acute presentations of ischaemic stroke and should be able to cope with the early complications after stroke. Emergency medical personnel should be trained to conduct a focused medical examination including the level of consciousness, the presence of focal weakness, the presence of seizure activity and the presence of aphasia and other major cognitive disturbances. They need to be informed about fluctuating or stuttering courses and that early clearing of symptoms is of special importance, and they need to learn about the complexity of stroke presentation and its differential diagnosis in order to understand why early involvement of specialists in this field is desirable. It is particularly essential for these groups to learn that they are important and competent partners in the team providing acute stroke care. The concept of 'time is brain' should be understood by all involved in the 'stroke chain'. No waste of time should be allowed when the patients have arrived at the hospital and written standards for in-hospital delays should be available in hospitals receiving patients with acute stroke. One example is that set by the National Institute of Neurological Disorders and Stroke in 1997 [National Institute of Neurological Disorders and Stroke, 1997].

Stroke as an Emergency

Stroke is a medical and occasionally also a surgical emergency. The success of care of the acute stroke victim begins with the recognition both by the public and the health professional that stroke is an emergency, like acute myocardial infarction (MI) and trauma. The majority of stroke patients do no receive thrombolytic therapy because they do not reach the hospital soon enough [Barber et al., 2001]. Successful care of the acute stroke victim as an emergency depends on a 4-step chain: (1) rapid recognition of and reaction to stroke warning signs, (2) immediate use of EMS, (3) priority transport with notification of the receiving hospital and (4) rapid and accurate diagnosis and treatment at the hospital.

Failure to recognize stroke symptoms, anosognosia, and inability to move without assistance, living alone, financial concerns and calling/consulting a doctor increase the interval between stroke onset and hospital arrival (level III) [Ferro et al., 1994; Derex et al., 2002; Harraf et al., 2002].

Once stroke symptoms are suspected, patients or their proxies should call the EMS. Ambulance transportation decreases the delay of arrival at the hospital after stroke onset (level III). Helicopter transport is playing an increasing role in interfacility transfer of patients with stroke and should be activated earlier [Thomas et al., 2002]. The EMS system should have an electronic validated algorithm of questions to diagnose stroke during the phone interview with the patient/proxy [Porteous et al., 1999; Camerlingo et al., 2001]. Patients with onset of stroke symptoms within less than 3 h should be given priority in evaluation/transportation by the EMS. The EMS ambulance dispatchers should be able to recognize stroke symptoms and signs [Kothari et al., 1995, 1997] (level III) and identify and provide appropriate help for patients who need emergent care because of impaired consciousness, seizures, vomiting, haemodynamic instability or other early complications or comorbidity of stroke. In the near future, optimal management of stroke patients may include the administration of neuroprotective medications in the pre-hospital setting.

Referral

Stroke patients should be treated in stroke units [Stroke Unit Trialists' Collaboration, 2002]. Suspected stroke victims should be transported without delay to the nearest medical centre with an available stroke unit. Such stroke units should work in co-operation with primary care physicians for primary and secondary prevention and management of late complications of stroke and with rehabilitation and long-term care facilities when available. In each community, a network of stroke units or, if stroke units are not yet available, a network of medical centres providing organized acute stroke care should be organized and publicized near the public, the health professionals and the emergency transport systems.

If a GP or other doctor receives a call or consults a patient with suspected stroke, he should recommend/arrange emergent transportation, preferably through the EMS system, to the nearest emergency room of a hospital providing organized acute stroke care or a stroke unit if available. The EMS ambulance dispatchers should inform the stroke unit personnel that they are going to refer a stroke patient and describe his/her clinical status.

The initial evaluation of stroke patients can be made by emergency room doctors. In fact, emergency room doctors can correctly make the diagnosis of stroke in about 90% of the cases [Ferro et al., 1998] (level III). Emergent management of acute stroke includes two parallel processes: (1) diagnosis and treatment of life-threatening comorbid conditions and complication of stroke and (2) medical and neurological evaluation and treatment of the stroke itself.

Patients with subarachnoid haemorrhage should be referred urgently to a hospital where neurosurgical treatment, neuroradiological interventions and neurointensive care are available (level I).

Recommendations

1. Stroke patients should be treated in stroke units (level I). Therefore, suspected stroke victims should be transported without delay to the nearest medical centre with an available stroke unit, or to a hospital providing organized acute stroke care if a stroke unit is not available.
2. Once stroke symptoms are suspected, patients or their proxies should call the EMS or a similar emergency medical system (level III).
3. Patients with subarachnoid haemorrhage should be referred urgently to a centre with facilities for neurosurgical treatment, neuroradiological interventions and neurointensive care (level I).

Emergency Management

The time window for treatment of patients with acute stroke is narrow. Acute emergency management of stroke therefore requires parallel processes at different levels of patient management. For example, acute assessment of neurological and vital functions parallels treatment of acutely life-threatening conditions. The selection of special treatment strategies may already be ongoing before the final decision on the subtype of acute stroke has been made. Time is the most important factor, especially the minutes and first hours after stroke onset.

The acute stroke patient, even the one with milder symptoms, must be recognized as an urgently ill medical patient [Brott et al., 1994; Brott and Reed, 1989; Adams et al., 1994]. The patient has to be transported to an emergency unit, and the examining physician must assess the stroke patient with the priority for a life-threatening and disabling illness. Of course, only a minority of the stroke patients present with an immediate life-threatening condition, but many have severe abnormalities in basic physiologic functions. One of the problems in the early treatment of acute stroke is to distinguish patients who need immediate life support and treatment in an intensive care unit from those who can be managed in a stroke unit or normal ward. Symptoms and signs which may predict later complications such a space-occupying infarction or bleeding, recurrent stroke, and medical conditions such as hypertensive crisis, co-existing MI, aspiration pneumonia and renal failure must be recognized early. Also, early assessment of stroke subtypes based on the physical and neurological evaluation as well as on skilled interpretation of neuroimaging is essential for the prediction of a high risk of early recurrence.

Initial Assessment in the Emergency Unit

The majority of stroke patients nowadays enter the hospital via the emergency or receiving unit. A different management strategy is necessary if the patient arrives at the hospital within the first few hours after stroke onset compared with patients who arrive later, for example 24 h after stroke. In the first case, the neurological examination has to be focused on the severity of deficits, lesion localization and possible sources of stroke. Simultaneously, conditions such as hypertensive crisis, elevated blood glucose, aspiration, seizures or cardiac arrhythmias must be recognized and treatment options considered. Time is critical since the therapeutic window for specific therapies may be quite narrow.

Written protocols for stroke are a prerequisite for standardized patient care. Printed checklists can be implemented to ensure that the protocols are used regularly. They should be produced for each stage in the management. These checklists should be formulated by the specialist co-ordinating stroke care in consultation with the team staff and include the types of possible interventions and specify the ranges of pathologically modified parameters for such interventions, e.g. elevated blood glucose levels or high blood pressure levels. The beneficial effect of in-hospital care pathways has not been firmly established by randomized trials [Kwan and Sandercock, 2003], but single reports have claimed that the use of protocols has been shown to significantly reduce the length of hospital stay and cost per patient as well as the incidence of complications [Odderson and McKenna, 1993].

Factors delaying early intervention within the hospital include (1) admission policies that require placement of patients in general medical wards, (2) lack of access to early brain-imaging facilities, (3) rating of stroke as non-urgent by hospital staff, (4) lack of treatment facilities for stroke and (5) unavailability of a neurologist or other physician with stroke expertise in the emergency room [Jørgensen et al., 1996; Wester et al., 1999].

The initial examination includes observation of breathing function, assessment of blood pressure and heart rate and determination of arterial oxygen saturation using infrared pulse oxymetry if available. Simultaneously, blood samples for clinical chemistry, coagulation and haematology studies are drawn and a venous line is inserted. Standard electrolyte solutions are given until clinical chemistry results are available. After the emergency assessment, which in part will be done by emergency nurses or other emergency room personnel, the neurologist should perform a targeted neurological examination. The examination is supplemented, if possible, by a careful medical history focusing on atherosclerotic risk factors and cardiac disease. Especially in young patients, a history of drug abuse, oral contraceptive use, infection, trauma or migraine may give important clues.

The initial goal is to distinguish a cerebral infarction from intracerebral or subarachnoid haemorrhage using CT imaging as soon as possible. Immediate imaging (CT or MRI) is mandatory particularly in candidates for thrombolysis.

Initial Emergent Treatment

Airways, Breathing and Pulmonary Function. Securing adequate oxygenation is an important part of general emergency procedures. In stroke patients, hypoxia may be caused by pre-existing pulmonary conditions, changes in the ventilatory drive or aspiration. Securing airways is of special importance in patients with reduced consciousness [Horner et al., 1988]. In acute ischaemic stroke, early changes in ventilatory drive and early respiratory disturbances due to reduced consciousness are rare. However, patients with complete hemispheric or middle cerebral artery (MCA) ischaemia, large supratentorial or infratentorial haemorrhage or brainstem stroke may develop early ventilatory problems. In those cases, an endotracheal tube should be considered [Grotta et al., 1995]. Therefore, it is mandatory that patients with severe stroke are continuously monitored with pulse oxymetry. They should be treated with supplemental oxygen, usually 2–4 litres per minute via nasal tubes for the acute period until the patient is stable, the diagnostic procedure is completed and the patient has been brought to the ward [Hacke et al., 1995]. Sleep apnoea is frequent during the first night after cerebral infarction (62%) and is associated with early neurologic worsening [Iranzo et al., 2002].

Concomitant Heart Disease. Cardiac abnormalities are frequently found with deep MCA infarcts, especially those involving the insular cortex. Nonetheless, the physician must carefully exclude acute MI and look for atrial fibrillation or valvular disease. Each of these disorders may predispose to stroke and may jeopardize cardiac function. Concomitant stroke and MI are a specifically serious problem and carry a bad prognosis. A significant percentage of elderly stroke patients may have low cardiac output at the time of stroke onset. The cardiac examination of the stroke patient includes assessment of the presence of tachypnoea, tachycardia, jugular venous distension, peripheral oedema or a third heart sound.

Antihypertensive Treatment in the Acute Phase

Acute stroke, either ischaemic or haemorrhagic, leads to a hypertensive reaction in the first hours and days after stroke. Most investigators nowadays agree that hypertension should not be treated drastically in the first hours after stroke. However, there are no data recommending thresholds or time points of intervention, and which drugs to use for hypertension control. Antihypertensive drugs should be used only in rare exceptions in the early hours following acute ischaemic stroke [Brott and Reed, 1989], i.e. for hypertensive crisis or heart failure if the systolic blood pressure exceeds 220 mm Hg on repeated measures or if the diastolic pressure exceeds 120 mm Hg [Adams et al., 1994]. Drugs recommended for the treatment of such elevated hypertension vary from country to country. In essence, short-acting parenteral drugs that may be titrated over a venous line can be controlled best [Hacke et al., 1995]. Sublingual nifedipine should be avoided.

In some stroke patients hypotension exists. This is of special risk in the setting of haemodynamic stenosis of intra- or extracranial vessels. Frequently, volume depletion is the cause of hypotension. Correction of hypovolaemia using hyperoncotic fluids and, in a few patients, also pressor drugs may be the treatment of choice.

Optimising Fluid and Electrolyte Balance. The main goal of fluid management in the acute phase is to establish and to maintain normovolaemia. Fluid depletion is best treated with isotonic saline or Ringer's solution. Glucose-containing infusions are best avoided if there is no hypoglycaemia. Proper fluid management is the basis for an optimal cardiac output, which is desirable in the basic treatment of acute stroke [Adams et al., 1994; Hacke et al., 1995; The European Ad Hoc Consensus Group, 1997].

Blood Glucose and Elevated Body Temperature. Experimentally, hyperglycaemia increases infarct size [Pulsinelli et al., 1983]. There are reports that a high glucose level at admission is linked to poorer neurological outcome after stroke. In some studies, the independent contribution of admission glucose levels to predict neurological outcome disappeared if acute-phase reaction markers such as the erythrocyte sedimentation rate were incorporated in multivariate predictor models [Chamorro et al., 1995]. No controlled data are available concerning blood glucose control following acute stroke. Nevertheless, since hyperglycaemia may either be part of the stress response after stroke or a sign of unrecognized diabetes, it seems to be advisable to include treatment of hyperglycaemia into the general treatment recommendations after stroke. Thresholds for intervention have not been prospectively established. In some centres, a cut-off value of >10 mmol/l blood glucose has been proposed. Elevated blood glucose should be counteracted using small doses of intravenous insulin. Since hypoglycaemia (<2.2 mmol/l) can also exacerbate neurological focal deficits, blood glucose levels must be measured in any patient presenting with symptoms and signs of acute stroke. Normalization of the blood glucose level using 20 g of oral glucose or 10% glucose infusion by peripheral vein or 20% glucose via central venous line may reverse neurological dysfunction due to hypoglycaemia [Adams et al., 1994; The European Ad Hoc Consensus Group, 1996]. Except for the treatment of hypoglycaemia, no glucose-containing infusions should be used in the early or unstable stroke patient. Elevated body temperature may also negatively influence stroke outcome [Reith et al., 1996; Castillo et al., 1998]. Lowering of elevated body temperature to normal is strongly suggested. But in spite of overwhelming experimental data and anecdotal clinical reports, this issue is not yet solved on the basis of randomized clinical experience.

Recommendations

1 Secure airways and give oxygen to patients with severe acute stroke (level III).
2 Do not treat hypertension in patients with ischaemic stroke if they do not have critically elevated blood pressure levels (level III).
3 Treat fever and lower elevated blood glucose (level III).

Imaging and Functional Tests

It is essential that all stroke patients after admittance in the emergency room are immediately investigated neurologically and with regard to vital functions (table 2). Time is critical since the therapeutic window may be quite narrow for specific treatment, both in patients with acute ischaemia and haemorrhage. Differentiation between the two can only be performed by brain imaging, and different types of ischaemic stroke need vascular studies in addition.

Cranial CT is widely available and reliably distinguishes not only between haemorrhage and ischaemic stroke or subarachnoid haemorrhage, but can also rule out other brain diseases. Signs of early ischaemia can sometimes be detected as early as 2 h after stroke onset, but this may be difficult even for the trained examiner, in particular in very early studies. Early infarct signs include sulcus effacement, swelling of the basal ganglia and the hyperintense MCA sign. Early signs of extensive infarction with intracranial midline shifts indicate a very serious event and a high risk, both for secondary haemorrhage and large malignant oedema formation and may hence need short-time repeated imaging.

Parenchymal haemorrhage can be identified almost immediately either in deep structures in patients with hypertension or in atypical areas, in patients without hypertension or under adequate treatment usually due to cerebral amyloid angiopathy. Infratentorial haemorrhage or cerebellar infarcts can be identified similarly to supratentorial lesions, but smaller haemorrhages/ischaemic infarcts in particular in the brainstem may easily be missed. In addition, CT may detect subarachnoid blood in the majority of cases with subarachnoid haemorrhage. Sometimes haemorrhages may even be interpreted as primary, but are indeed secondary to ischaemic events: involvement of vascular territories are always indicative of such conditions, which are easier to identify in MRI studies. Brain haemorrhages tend to grow in the first 6–12 h after stroke in about 40–50% of all patients even without clinical deterioration, which makes a second early CT study necessary, in particular if patients deteriorate. CT angiography (CTA) is a reliable tool to obtain information on extra- and intracranial arterial patency, and its use in clinical practice often adds value to the diagnostic workup [Schellinger et al., 2003].

MRI is more sensitive and is increasingly used in referral hospitals with stroke unit expertise as a standard procedure. Recent objections because of a suspected lower sensitivity to identify brain haemorrhages were over-

Table 2. Emergent diagnostic tests in acute stroke

1	CT
2	ECG and chest X-ray
3	Clinical chemistry
	a Complete blood count and platelet count, prothrombin time, INR, PTT
	b Serum electrolytes
	c Blood glucose
	d CRP, sedimentation rate
	e Arterial blood gas analysis, if hypoxia is suspected
	f Hepatic and renal chemical analyses
4	Pulse oxymetry
5	Lumbar puncture (negative CT and suspicion of subarachnoidal haemorrhage only)
6	Duplex and transcranial ultrasound
7	EEG if seizures are suspected
8	MRI and MRA in selected cases; CTA
9	Diffusion MR and perfusion MR in selected cases
10	Echocardiography (transthoracic and transoesophageal) in selected cases

INR = International normalized ratio; PTT = partial thromboplastin time; CRP = C-reactive protein.

come by modern MRI techniques such as T_2*-weighted imaging, which indeed are even more sensitive than CT scanning for the display of intracerebral haemorrhage. Diffusion MRI is very sensitive for early detection of the damaged brain tissue and combined with perfusion MRI may help identifying patients who benefit from early thrombolysis. In fact, current concepts suggest that patients with a significant perfusion-diffusion mismatch may benefit from restoration of the ischaemic penumbra surrounding an already necrotic core of infarction, whereas those with overlapping areas of diffusion and perfusion deficits have a less favourable benefit/risk ratio. However, these MR techniques are not yet available on a large scale but do seem promising tools for future routine applications. MR angiography (MRA) can be used to identify obliterations in the major intracranial arteries, but should carefully be interpreted if studies from extracranial cerebral arteries are missing. In this case, ultrasound can be useful to identify severe haemodynamically relevant carotid obstructions, which are likely to produce significant perfusion deficits in small embolic or lacunar strokes and may thus falsely mimic a remarkable perfusion-diffusion mismatch. MRA also plays a role in evaluating the venous system and aneurysms down to a diameter of 3 mm.

Ultrasound studies are routinely performed in stroke centres. The major goal is to identify large obstructive lesions in the extracranial as well as in the intracranial basal arteries. In addition, transcranial Doppler may be useful to monitor spontaneous or drug-induced thrombolysis in the majority of patients. In about one quarter of the patients, it is not possible or very difficult to insonate through small temporal bone windows without application of contrast agents. The detection of some causes, such as dissections, intimal hyperplasia and other less frequent aetiologies is facilitated by the systematic use of ultrasound studies. Transoesophageal and transthoracic echocardiography is frequently indicated in suspected cardioembolic stroke, but is usually not performed on an emergency basis. It seems useful to have these studies available within the first 24 h after onset of stroke to choose the best available secondary prevention, in particular in the presence of cardiac sources of embolism. They can also sometimes be identified by means of MCA monitoring if high-intensity transient signals are observed.

Recommendations

1 A head CT is the most important diagnostic tool in patients with suspected stroke to differentiate between ischaemia and haemorrhage.
2 Vascular imaging (ultrasound, CTA and MRA) in the acute condition gives additional information about the vessel patency in the brain and neck vessels and should supplement all imaging procedures already in the acute phase.
3 MRI/MRA can replace CT if performed appropriately, and in particular T_2*-weighted imaging is necessary to identify even small haemorrhages.
4 Diffusion and perfusion MRI may be of additional help for assessing the risk/benefit ratio for early revascularization therapy.

Stroke Units

Stroke care should take place in a stroke unit. A meta-analysis by the Stroke Unit Trialists' Collaboration [Stroke Unit Trialists' Collaboration, 2002] showed an 18% relative reduction in mortality, a reduction in death or dependence and a reduction in death or need of institutional care when treated in a stroke unit in comparison with a general medical ward (level I). The absolute changes indicated a 3% reduction in all-cause mortality (number needed to treat 33), a 3% reduction in the need for nursing home care, and a 6% increase in the number of independent survivors (number needed to treat 16). All types of patients with stroke benefit from treatment and rehabilitation in stroke units: males and females, young and elderly stroke patients and patients with mild, moderate and severe strokes.

Table 3. Requirements

Minimum requirements for centres managing acute stroke patients	
1	Availability of 24-hour CT scanning
2	Established stroke treatment guidelines and operational procedures
3	Close co-operation of neurologists, internists and rehabilitation experts
4	Specially trained nursing personnel
5	Early multidisciplinary rehabilitation including speech therapy, occupational therapy and physical therapy
6	Established network of rehabilitation facilities to provide a continuous process of care
7	Neurosonological investigations within 24 h (extracranial vessels, colour-coded duplex sonography)
8	ECG, echocardiography
9	Laboratory examinations (including coagulation parameters)
10	Monitoring of blood pressure, ECG, oxygen saturation, blood glucose, body temperature
Additional facilities recommended	
1	MRI/MRA
2	Diffusion and perfusion MR
3	CTA
4	Echocardiography (transoesophageal)
5	Cerebral angiography
6	Transcranial Doppler sonography
7	Specialized neuroradiological, neurosurgical and vascular surgical consultation

A stroke unit consists of a hospital unit or part of a hospital unit that exclusively or nearly exclusively takes care of stroke patients. A survey across Europe showed that various forms of stroke unit care exist [Brainin et al., 2000]. Most of such stroke units have in common that they provide a co-ordinated multidisciplinary approach to treatment and care. The core disciplines of such a multidisciplinary team are: medical treatment, nursing, physiotherapy, occupational therapy, speech and language therapy and social work. The multidisciplinary team should have a specialist interest in stroke management and work in a co-ordinated way (through regular meetings to plan patient care). Programmes of regular staff education and training should be provided.

The typical components of care in the stroke unit trials [Langhorne et al., 2002] were as follows: (a) assessment – medical assessment and diagnosis including CT scanning, early assessment of nursing and therapy needs; (b) early management policies – early mobilization, prevention of complications (e.g. pressure area care, careful positioning and handling) treatment of hypoxia, hyperglycaemia, pyrexia and dehydration, and (c) ongoing rehabilitation policies (co-ordinated multidisciplinary team care, early assessments of needs after discharge).

Stroke units are described in several categories: (1) acute stroke unit admitting patients acutely and continuing treatment for several days but usually less than 1 week; (2) comprehensive stroke unit admitting patients acutely and continuing treatment and rehabilitation for several weeks if necessary; (3) rehabilitation stroke unit admitting patients after a delay of 1 or 2 weeks and continuing treatment and rehabilitation for several weeks or months if necessary, and (4) a mobile stroke team is a mobile team offering stroke care and treatment to stroke patients at a variety of wards. Such teams are usually established in hospitals where stroke units are not available. Of these, only the comprehensive stroke unit and the rehabilitation stroke unit have proven effectiveness in terms of reduced mortality and handicap [Stroke Unit Trialists' Collaboration, 2002].

The optimal size of a stroke unit is not known, but should be adequate to provide specialist multidisciplinary stroke unit care for the whole duration of hospital admission. In practice, this is often achieved with a single comprehensive unit (in smaller hospitals) or a combination of acute unit and rehabilitation units (in larger hospitals). Further evidence is needed to recommend type and size of the most effective stroke units in more detail. Table 3 indicates the minimal requirements for centres managing acute stroke patients and additional recommended facilities.

Recommendations

1. Stroke patients should be treated in specialized stroke units (level I).
2. Stroke units should provide co-ordinated multidisciplinary care provided by medical, nursing and therapy staff who specialize in stroke care (level I).

Quality Management and Control of Process Quality

It is mandatory to establish a documentation system for all strokes in a way that allows to evaluate major characteristics of the patients treated in stroke units and to compare the results with other, similar units. Items chosen must also allow case mix analyses across units, regions or even countries. These should include major predictors of outcome such as age, NIH scale values at onset and diabetes. Several systems of documentations have been developed and recommended for use. It is important to

Table 4. Recommendations for the quality control of time frames for treatment of acute stroke

Time frame prolonged	Recommendation
Time from stroke onset to calling emergency service	Increase public information and support stroke awareness campaigns
Time from stroke onset to hospital door	Training of paramedics necessary
Time from hospital door to CT	Screening and revision of intra-hospital organization

make young colleagues understand that such documentations have to be performed concurrently by either the treating physicians or the stroke nurses themselves and should not be left to additional staff that otherwise does not participate in the work of the stroke unit. It is essential to have follow-up data at least 3 months following the stroke onset in order to enable benchmarking. These data should at least include mortality and Rankin Scale scores. In addition, process quality should also be monitored and evaluated on a regular basis. Some recommendations are listed in table 4.

Rehabilitation

More than half of the stroke patients in some Western countries are older than 75 years [Johansson, 2000]. One third of the stroke patients are younger, two thirds older than 65 years of age [Kaste et al., 1998]. Approximately 10% of stroke survivors are without disability and are able to function independently. Another 10% of patients are institutionalized because of markedly severe disability and are unable to achieve functional independence in a home setting. The remaining 80% of stroke survivors have mild to moderately severe disability and benefit most from rehabilitation [Joint Committee for Stroke Facilities, 1972]. Rehabilitation can reduce the number of patients who are left dependent after stroke.

Early Rehabilitation

Forty percent of stroke patients need active rehabilitation services. Rehabilitation of a stroke victim is started as soon as possible. This means that the patient should immediately be brought to a hospital with such facilities not only because of acute diagnosis and therapy but also because of early rehabilitation. Rehabilitation will be started as soon as he/she is clinically stable. The intensity of the actual rehabilitation program depends on the status of the patient and the degree of the disability. Whenever necessary (as in patients not capable of active training), passive methods should be used to prevent contractions and joint pain and to prevent distress for the patient when movement is restarted after immobilization. With passive rehabilitation, one can also minimize the risk of bedsores and pneumonia. All joints on the paralyzed side are moved through the full range of motion several times a day (3–4 times at least). When the patient recovers consciousness and is able to co-operate or if the patient has a normal level of consciousness already from the onset of symptoms, then he/she is encouraged to take an active part in the rehabilitation programme. Prolonged immobilization and hemiplegia carry the risk of deep venous thrombosis and the complication of pulmonary embolism. In hemiplegic patients and those stroke patients who must be immobile for more than a day or two, low-molecular-weight heparin therapy should be given subcutaneously. After 2 or 3 days, most patients who are alert can be moved out of bed with safety and placed in either a wheelchair or fixed chair for a good part of each day.

Effects of Acute Stroke Rehabilitation

The role of rehabilitative efforts has been widely recognized as being essential in the acute stage of stroke. The beneficial effects of rehabilitation-type stroke units have been well documented [Indredavik et al., 1991; Kalra and Eade, 1995]. Treatment of acute stroke patients in stroke units has been shown to reduce mortality, length of hospital stay, discharge rate to nursing homes and cost [Jørgensen et al., 1995, 1999, 2000]. Functional recovery has been significantly greater and more rapid in a stroke unit compared with general wards [Kalra and Eade, 1995]. Treatment in stroke units has increased the proportion of patients able to live at home long after their stroke [Indredavik et al., 1999]. Treatment in wards dedicated to stroke rehabilitation is based on multidisciplinary teamwork consisting of a physician, physiotherapist, speech therapist, occupational therapist, neuropsychologist, social worker and nurse [Stroke Unit Trialists' Collaboration, 2002]. In a functioning unit, there is a motivating and encouraging attitude that maintains a patient's own desire to improve. Important is a milieu of 'enriched environment', where patients feel comfortable and which supports the patient's efforts and encourages him/her to practise even beyond working hours [Johansson, 2000]. Elderly stroke patients may equally benefit from the well-organized management of stroke [Kaste et al., 1995; Jørgensen et al., 2000].

Unfortunately, many hospitals treating stroke patients do not have all these specially trained stroke experts. The core of the stroke team, physician, nurse, physiotherapist and speech therapist, can be found in most hospitals and they can provide a decent rehabilitation programme if they take it as a challenge.

Not all stroke patients do have an identical potential for recovery. Old age alone is no reason to exclude a patient from an effective rehabilitation programme. Indicators of neurological dysfunction are used to predict outcome and are valid for large groups of patients. For individual patients, the variation in outcome may still be larger. In view of this, it is generally recommended that the rehabilitation programme should be carried out in such borderline cases in order to assess a patient's potential for becoming independent. It is particularly rewarding when a patient who is believed to have no rehabilitation potential responds to treatment and becomes drastically less dependent.

Rehabilitation Programme

Once the initial phase of stroke has passed, the patients should be carefully assessed for the degree of disability and a detailed rehabilitation programme for him/her should be made. The assessment of the patient's situation includes evaluation of intellectual impairment including specific cognitive deficits such as aphasia, agnosia, apraxia, mood, motivation, the degree of motor weakness and sensory and visual loss.

After the assessment of a stroke patient by the members of the stroke rehabilitation team, a rehabilitation programme will be tailored according to the individual needs of the patient. Before the start of rehabilitation programme, every patient is carefully evaluated. In a meeting of the rehabilitation group, where a target of rehabilitation is set, the therapies used for this target are determined and explained also to the patient in detail. Patients with mild neurologic impairments, such as moderate hemiparesis, hemihypo-aesthesia, slightly reduced balance or mild to moderate cognitive deficits require only limited training in basic self-care, ambulation and functional communication. Subacute rehabilitation, consisting of 1–3 h of daily individual and group therapy, is considered appropriate for these patients. These recommendations are mostly based on clinical experience and expert consensus. Compelling evidence on the basis of randomized clinical data is not available for such patients nor for patients who have more severe impairments, such as hemiplegia with spasticity, visual-perceptual deficits, complex aphasia, dysphagia or multiple medical comorbidities. These patients are best managed in a subacute rehabilitation unit or should be admitted to a specialized rehabilitation hospital. In these settings, rehabilitation should be a full-day work. For patients with complex stroke syndromes, rehabilitation in a specialized ward or hospital is more efficient and cost effective than subacute rehabilitation at general medical wards or even in a nursing home [Kramer et al., 1997].

Especially cognitive and emotional disturbances are a challenging area for neurological rehabilitation. These domains are often underdiagnosed and underrecognized and should be a regular part of any rehabilitation programme for stroke patients. Recent recommendations have shown the beneficial effects as well as the efficacy of a number of techniques applied for disturbances of language, spatial perception, attention, memory, calculation and praxis [Cappa et al., 2003].

The progress of the patient needs to be followed on a daily basis by the different members involved. At regular conferences, at least in weekly or biweekly intervals, all members of the stroke team should meet and analyse the progress of individual stroke patients and compare them with the pre-specified goals that have been set up for this patient. Should there be a blocking in any of the aspects of the rehabilitation programme, the reason for this – for example untreated depression – needs to be found out and corrected, if possible. Not only the individual patients but also their carers and spouses should be involved into the rehabilitation process as early as possible. They should be instructed about the principles of stroke rehabilitation. The members of the family also need to be taught when not to help the patient in order to optimize the progress of the rehabilitation plan. As soon as the patient's condition allows, he/she should visit his/her own home to smooth the transit from hospital to home and increase the patients' motivation. The occupational therapist or a physiotherapist should undertake the home visit together with the patient to evaluate the changes needed at home in order to support the patient's discharge from hospital [Kaste et al., 1995].

As soon as it is obvious that the patient needs a longer rehabilitation period than can be provided within the acute hospital, he/she should be transferred to a special rehabilitation ward or a rehabilitation hospital wherever available. When the patient is transferred to a rehabilitation hospital, it is of the utmost importance that all members of the stroke team transfer documentation of the patient's progress to the stroke team of the rehabilitation hospital [Kaste et al., 1995]. After institutional rehabilitation, the rehabilitation programme can be taken over by an out-patient rehabilitation clinic. This ensures the smooth transfer of the patient to the next rehabilitation step back to normal. The length of the rehabilitation period in the acute stage depends upon the severity of the stroke and locally available stroke rehabilitation services. Under usual circumstances, rehabilitation following the acute phase of ischaemic stroke should not last longer than 6–12 weeks and rarely more than 24 weeks.

Developing Methods of Stroke Rehabilitation

A challenge for stroke rehabilitation is to determine exactly which components of co-ordinated care lead to better outcomes, so that maximum improvement can be delivered in a cost-effective manner. Brain research has produced new information that gives encouraging insight into rehabilitation after stroke and helps to develop new techniques. Recent reports of rehabilitation methods that are based on developing muscle strength and increasing the width of movements with plentiful repetition and enhanced resistance training of the affected limb are called 'forced use'. Novel restorative programmes that focus on the functional improvement of the upper extremity [Taub et al., 1993; Miltner et al., 1999] or on the recovery of gait [Hesse et al., 1996; Hesse, 2001; Werner et al., 2002] have provided promising tools for the treatment of stroke patients with residual disability. It is thought that these techniques are based on the principles of plasticity in the adult human brain which allow the re-organization of nervous networks. This plasticity can be activated by repeated task-specific training.

The interventions that have been shown to be effective require active participation of the patient, repetitive training and a lot of practice and often involve resistant training. A critical re-examination of the current assumptions underlying traditional facilitatory approaches is needed [Duncan, 1997].

Late Rehabilitation

The fastest recovery of neurological deficit occurs during the first 3 months after the onset of symptoms. This is also the optimal time for rehabilitation. Active rehabilitation, however, should be administrated as long as objective improvement in the neurological function is observed. Returning to the community can be a traumatic experience to the stroke patient and various support services have been developed beyond primary health care to enhance coping with the illness and to facilitate return to normal life. In addition to national organizations involved in providing information to stroke survivors, the role of locally based self-help groups is important in supporting stroke patients and their caregivers. The general opinion is, however, that there is a low level of service provision especially for older stroke survivors living in the community, and more rehabilitation and co-operation with primary and secondary health care would be required to ensure an optimal long-term outcome.

Since most elderly patients prefer to stay at home, community care has acquired a greater relevance. An important requirement of good health care and social services for older people living in the community would be flexibility of service provision, implying the need for patient assessment before admission to the appropriate service [Black and Bowman, 1997]. A well-integrated social and medical care with case management programmes may be one way to reduce admission to institutions and prevent the functional decline in the elderly [Bernabei et al., 1998].

Aspects of Home Treatment in the Chronic Phase of Stroke

After most of the improvement in neurological dysfunction has occurred and the active rehabilitation programme has come to an end, the stroke patient needs a long-term rehabilitation programme. This is to guarantee that the functional status which has been achieved during the acute rehabilitation programme is sustained. Should the functional outcome of a patient be in jeopardy and an active comprehensive rehabilitation programme is needed, it is sometimes reasonable to re-admit the patient for a more intensive in-patient rehabilitation period. A decision concerning the duration of out-patient therapy is based upon therapy objectives. A major goal for the patient and his/her family is to acquire ambulation as independently as possible, also in patients with hemiplegia, and to achieve an optimal level for the activities of daily living. Once such techniques of unaided self-help have been learned, regular, intensive therapy can be discontinued. Criteria for re-instituting therapy is based on a change in the patient's function, either deterioration or improvement [Reding and McDowell, 1987]. For speech therapy, the end point should be patient performance. When the patient's function reach a plateau and no significant gains are seen, formal therapy should be discontinued. By this time, it is hoped that patient and family will have been instructed adequately in speech and language techniques focused on the patient's needs. The patient and family should continue working together on these problems on a daily basis.

Of utmost importance is that a patient has somebody for his/her support, either a spouse or some other caregiver. Self-esteem, empowerment and social competence are indispensable factors of success. Most essential in long-term stroke rehabilitation is that the patient and his/her family assume responsibility for the further continuation of the rehabilitation programme. Without the patient's own desire to maintain or even improve the abilities of daily living and social functioning, any attempts of rehabilitation workers become vastly more difficult. Supporting the patient in his/her social environment is important. Keeping up social contacts is perhaps something that offers the best opportunity to influence the patient's quality of life. Every chronic stroke patient with a marked disability should have regular contact with a family physician, who can encourage the patient, notice possible impairment of clinical state and take care of secondary prevention.

Assessment of the Quality of Rehabilitation

The results of the rehabilitation programme for patients with stroke should be measured by means of appropriate assessment scales. Most important are those that assess whether the patient can return home or is institutionalized on the basis of achieved self-care abilities and independence in activities of daily living. One useful and widely used scale is the Barthel Index [Mahoney and Barthel, 1965] and, more recently, the Functional Independence Measure [Granger et al., 1994]. The walking ability, functional ambulatory classification [Holden et al., 1984] and the speed of gait [Wade et al., 1987] give an idea about the patient's ambulation ability. For the quality of life assessment, no universally accepted scale for use in stroke patients has evolved so far. This also applies for dementia and for depression after stroke, which are common events following stroke. For depression, several rating scales have been in use, one being the Montgomery-Asberg Depression Rating Scale [Montgomery and Åsberg, 1979], which is short and easy to apply, however relevant with good validity. Measures of recovery should not only focus on sensorimotor function domains but also on cognitive and emotional aspects. Clinical experience shows that impairment in attentional components, factors relating to semantic memory, word fluency and spatial orientation are strongly associated with attainment of independent ambulation and self-care. In addition, emotional factors are associated with every success and failure and cover a wide range. They include hope for emotional devotion and sexual desires.

Is There Evidence that Rehabilitation Programmes Are Indicated?

With focused rehabilitation programmes, stroke patients can become ambulatory and largely independent. Of major importance is that the majority of survivors are able to live at home and do not require nursing home care. A controlled, randomized study from Helsinki compared patients who were treated and rehabilitated systematically by a stroke team with patients included in a less systematic stroke management programme trial [Kaste et al., 1995]. The results showed that elderly stroke patients treated by a stroke team were able to leave the hospital on an average 16 days earlier (24 vs. 40 days), went directly home more often (75 vs. 62%) and were more often fully independent in activities of daily living (76 vs. 59%) 1 year after the onset of stroke. A better outcome of stroke is of benefit in both human and economic terms. That such results can be achieved with systematic stroke management and not by a chance is verified by identical results from University Hospitals of Umeå, Sweden [Strand et al., 1985], Copenhagen, Denmark [Jørgensen et al., 1995], Kuopio, Finland [Sivenius et al., 1985] and Trondheim, Norway [Indredavik et al., 1991].

Recommendations

1 Every patient should have access to evaluation for rehabilitation.
2 In patients with a clear indication for rehabilitation, treatment should be initiated early after stroke (level I). Disabled patients should have access to structured care including institutional care.
3 Rehabilitation should be provided by a multidisciplinary team in a stroke unit (level I).
4 Intensity and duration of rehabilitation should be optimal for each patient; new methods of rehabilitation should be used (e.g. repetitive training and forced use), ideally supplementary to established methods (level IV).
5 Patients with chronic symptomatic stroke should be supported in their social environment. This includes access to a family physician, evaluation of out-patient rehabilitation services, secondary prevention and support in psychosocial functioning (level II).

---

high prevalence of environmental exposure, a small increase in the RR of stroke due to environmental tobacco smoke may be associated with a great attributable risk in the community [Wells, 1994]. After adjusting for age, gender, BP, heart disease and DM, there is a 1.82-fold increased risk of stroke [95% confidence interval (CI): 1.3–2.5] in non-smokers and long-term ex-smokers with environmental tobacco exposure [Wolf et al., 1988].

Alcohol Consumption

The association between alcohol consumption and stroke is complex and may differ between Caucasian and other populations, e.g. Japanese people. In the Honolulu Heart Program, heavy drinkers had a three times higher risk of haemorrhagic stroke (subarachnoid haemorrhage or intracerebral haemorrhage) than non-drinkers [Donahue et al., 1986]. A case-control study in a multiethnic population suggested that moderate consumption (up to 2 drinks of spirits, 2 cans of beer or 2 glasses of wine, equivalent to 20–30 g of ethyl alcohol per day) was associated with a decreased risk of ischaemic stroke, while heavy alcohol consumption is associated with an increased risk of ischaemic and haemorrhagic stroke [Goldstein et al., 2001]. A recent meta-analysis has given similar results by showing that heavy alcohol drinking (more than 60 g/day) increases the RR of stroke, while light or moderate alcohol consumption may be protective against total and ischaemic stroke [Reynolds et al., 2003]: a consumption of less than 12 g of alcohol per day was associated with a reduced risk of total stroke (RR = 0.83) and ischaemic stroke (RR = 0.80) and a moderate consumption of alcohol (12–24 g/day) was associated with a reduced RR of ischaemic stroke, 0.72 [Reynolds et al., 2003].

Lifestyle Modifications

Physical activity is inversely related with the risk of stroke [Lee et al., 1999]. However, this association has not been as extensively studied as the relationship between physical activity and CHD. A recent prospective cohort study of men participating in the Physician Health Study has revealed that exercise vigorous enough to work up a sweat was associated with a decreased risk of stroke [Lee et al., 1999]: the data suggested that this association was mediated through beneficial effects on body weight, BP, serum cholesterol and glucose tolerance, and that, apart from these effects, physical activity had no influence on stroke incidence.

Modifying diet reduces the risk of ischaemic heart disease and probably stroke: substantial evidence supports the use of diets high in non-hydrogenated unsaturated fats, whole grains, fruit and vegetables and adequate omega-3 fatty acids [Hu and Willett, 2002]. Eating fish once a month may also be associated with a decreased risk of stroke in men [He et al., 2002]. Such a diet should be low in salt and saturated fat.

Postmenopausal Oestrogen Replacement Therapy

Stroke rates rise rapidly in women once they become menopausal. However, in an analysis based on a 16-year follow-up of 59,337 postmenopausal women participating in the Nurses' Health Study, there was only a weak association between stroke and oestrogen replacement [Grodstein et al., 2001]. According to the recent HERS II trial, hormone replacement in healthy postmenopausal women is associated with an increased risk of ischaemic stroke [Grady et al., 2002].

Recommendations

1. BP measurement is an essential component of regular health care visits. BP should be lowered to normal levels (<140/<90 mm Hg or <135/80 mm Hg in diabetics) by means of lifestyle modification. Most hypertensive patients will also need pharmacological treatment to achieve normal BP (level I).
2. Although strict control of glucose levels in DM has not been proven to be associated with a decreased risk of stroke, it should be encouraged because of benefits in terms of other diabetic complications (level III).
3. Cholesterol-lowering therapy (simvastatin) is recommended for high-risk patients (level I).
4. Cigarette smoking should be discouraged (level II).
5. Heavy use of alcohol should be discouraged, light or moderate alcohol consumption may be protective against stroke (level I).
6. Regular physical activity is recommended (level II).
7. A low salt, low saturated fat, high fruit and vegetable diet rich in fibre is recommended (level II).
8. Subjects with an elevated body mass index should take a weight-reducing diet (level II).
9. Hormone replacement therapy (oestrogen/progestagen) should not be used for primary prevention of stroke (level I).

Antithrombotic Therapy

In Low- or Medium-Risk Patients

Six large randomised controlled trials have assessed aspirin in the primary prevention of vascular events [Peto et al., 1988; Steering Committee of the Physicians' Health Study Research Group, 1989; ETDRS Investigators, 1992; Hansson et al., 1998; Meade, 1998; de Gaetano, 2001]. A meta-analysis assessed data from the first 5 of these trials comparing aspirin with no aspirin in 52,251 subjects [Hart et al., 2000a]: after a mean follow-up of 4.6 years, the average stroke rate was 0.3% per year. Whilst aspirin reduced the risk of MI (RR: 0.74; 95% CI: 0.68–

0.82), it had no effect on stroke (RR: 1.08; 95% CI: 0.95–1.24).

The Primary Prevention Project Trial assessed aspirin (100 mg per day) and vitamin E in a factorial trial in 4,495 people with one or more of the following risk factors: hypertension, hypercholesterolaemia, DM, obesity, family history of premature MI or older age [de Gaetano, 2001]. After a mean follow-up of 3.6 years, aspirin had reduced total cardiovascular events by 29%; a non-significant reduction in stroke by 33% was also apparent.

Taken together, this study [de Gaetano, 2001] and the meta-analysis [Hart et al., 2000a] do not provide evidence supporting the use of aspirin for stroke prevention in healthy persons and in subjects at low or moderate vascular risk. Nevertheless, aspirin does reduce MI in subjects at moderate risk and can be recommended in those with one or more vascular risk factors [de Gaetano, 2001; Hart et al., 2000a]. No data are available on the use of other antithrombotic agents such as clopidogrel, ticlopidine or dipyridamole in primary prevention of stroke.

In Patients with High-Grade Asymptomatic Internal Carotid Artery Stenosis

Only one trial has been conducted in asymptomatic stenosis of the internal carotid artery (ICA): 372 patients with a stenosis of more than 50% were randomised between aspirin 325 mg per day and placebo [Côté et al., 1995]. The primary end point was any vascular event (TIA, cerebral infarct, MI, unstable angina or vascular death). After 2.3 years of follow-up, no difference appeared between both groups. However, the number of events was small and the trial had limited statistical power. Therefore, although there is no evidence that aspirin is beneficial in patients with asymptomatic ICA stenosis, if these patients are at an increased risk of MI, there is a consensus to use aspirin.

In Patients with Atrial Fibrillation

Atrial fibrillation (AF) is associated with a high rate of ischaemic stroke, the risk being similar whether AF is sustained or paroxysmal/intermittent [Hart et al., 2000b]. The average stroke rate was 5% per year in patients randomised to the control group of primary prevention trials [Lip and Lowe, 1996; Laupacis et al., 1998]. However, this rate varies substantially among subpopulations of AF patients ranging from 0.5 up to 12% per year [Lip and Lowe 1996; Laupacis et al., 1998].

Oral anticoagulation markedly decreases the risk of stroke in patients with AF, as found in 5 primary prevention trials [Petersen et al., 1989; The Stroke Prevention in Atrial Fibrillation Investigators, 1992; The Boston Area Anticoagulation Trial for Atrial Fibrillation Investigators 1990; Connolly et al., 1991; Ezekowitz et al., 1992; Stroke Prevention in Atrial Fibrillation Investigators 1994; SPAF III Writing Committee for the Stroke Prevention in Atrial Fibrillation Investigators, 1998; Hart et al., 1998]. A meta-analysis of these trials found that oral anticoagulation with warfarin reduced the rate of ischaemic stroke by 70% as compared with untreated patients. Assessment of the optimal intensity of anticoagulation in the European Atrial Fibrillation Trial, a secondary prevention trial, showed that anticoagulation to the international normalised ratio (INR) level of between 2.0 and 2.9 reduced the combined incidence of ischaemic and haemorrhagic events by 80% when compared with an INR of below 2.0, i.e. there was no reduction in thromboembolic events when INR levels were below 2.0 [The European Atrial Fibrillation Study Group, 1995]. An INR between 3.0 and 3.9 reduced total stroke rate by 40% [The European Atrial Fibrillation Study Group, 1995]. The risk of bleeding complications became substantial when the INR exceeded 5.0 [The European Atrial Fibrillation Study Group, 1995].

Aspirin (325 mg per day) was assessed in 4 randomised trials involving patients with AF and reduced stroke by 21% as compared with placebo [Hart et al., 1998]. In 2 of these trials, aspirin was significantly less efficacious than warfarin [Hart et al., 1998]. In the SPAF III trial, the combination of fixed dose warfarin (0.4–3.0 mg per day to raise the INR to between 1.2 and 1.5) and aspirin (325 mg per day) was ineffective in preventing stroke in AF patients [SPAF III Writing Committee for the Stroke Prevention in Atrial Fibrillation Investigators, 1998].

As the annual rate of stroke among people with AF is very wide, risk stratification should be used to determine whether patients are given anticoagulation, aspirin or nothing. Several risk stratification schemes have been published, e.g. by the Atrial Fibrillation Investigators and the SPAF group, and are broadly comparable [Laupacis et al., 1998]. Patients with AF who have one or more risk factors – previous stroke, TIA or systemic embolism, age over 75 years, arterial hypertension or left ventricular dysfunction – are at high risk of embolic stroke and should be offered anticoagulation (target INR of 2.5, range 2.0–3.0) unless this is contraindicated [Laupacis et al., 1998]. Patients over 65 years without other risk factors may be considered at moderate risk and either warfarin or aspirin (325 mg per day) may be appropriate according to the patient's wishes [Laupacis et al., 1998]. Younger patients with AF and no other cardiovascular disease ('lone AF') are at lowest risk of cardio-embolism and should be treated with aspirin or nothing, again according to their wishes [Laupacis et al., 1998].

Contraindications to warfarin include poor compliance, uncontrolled hypertension, small vessel disease on computed tomography (CT) or magnetic resonance imaging, alcohol dependency, liver disease, epilepsy, recurrent falls, bleeding lesions (peptic ulcer, previous cerebral haemorrhage) or tendency to bleeding (including coagulation defects, thrombocytopenia) [Lip and Lowe, 1996]. In this case, aspirin can be considered [Fuster et al., 2001].

The risk of embolic stroke is increased in patients with all prosthetic heart valves. Patients with mechanical valves have a higher risk than subjects with tissue valves. Anticoagulation has been proven effective for preventing stroke in this situation. Long-term anticoagulation is recommended for patients with AF who have mitral valve disease or prosthetic heart valves (mechanical or tissue valves). The target intensity of anticoagulation should be based on the particular type of prosthesis, but not less than INR 2–3 [Fuster et al., 2001].

Recommendations

1 Although aspirin does not reduce the risk of stroke in healthy subjects, it does reduce the risk of MI and can be recommended in subjects with one or more vascular risk factors (level I).
2 Clopidogrel, ticlopidine, trifusal and dipyridamole have not been studied in asymptomatic subjects and therefore cannot be recommended for primary stroke prevention (level IV).
3 Asymptomatic patients with an ICA stenosis of more than 50% should receive aspirin in order to reduce the risk of MI (level IV).
4 Long-term oral anticoagulation therapy (target INR 2.5; range 2.0–3.0) should be considered for all AF patients at high risk of embolism: age >75 years, or age >60 years plus risk factors such as high BP, left ventricular dysfunction or DM (level I).
5 Long-term aspirin (325 mg per day) or warfarin should be considered for patients with non-valvular AF at moderate risk for embolism: age 60–75 years without additional risk factors (level I).
6 Warfarin should be considered for AF patients aged 60–75 with DM or CHD (level I).
7 Although not yet established by randomised studies, in patients over 75 years, warfarin may be used with a lower INR (target INR of 2.0; range 1.6–2.5) to decrease the risk of haemorrhage (level III).
8 Patients with AF unable to receive oral anticoagulants should be offered aspirin (level I).
9 Long-term aspirin (325 mg per day) or no therapy should be considered for patients with non-valvular AF at low risk for embolism: age <60 years without additional risk factors (level I).
10 Patients with AF who have prosthetic heart valves should receive long-term anticoagulation with a target INR based on the prosthesis type, but not less than INR 2–3 (level II).

Carotid Surgery for Asymptomatic Carotid Stenosis

The prevalence of asymptomatic stenosis of the ICA in older people (age >65 years) is 10% in men and 5–7% in women [Fine-Edelstein et al., 1994]. Observational studies, long-term follow-up and data from patients in the NASCET and ECST trials (patients with asymptomatic stenosis contralateral to the operated symptomatic ICA) show a yearly stroke rate of 2–3% [Norris et al., 1991; European Carotid Surgery Trialists Collaborative Group, 1995; Inzitari et al., 2000; Nadareishvili et al., 2002; Sacco, 2001].

The results of 4 trials assessing carotid surgery in asymptomatic patients are still a matter of controversy. The largest of these trials, the Asymptomatic Carotid Atherosclerosis Study, reported that patients with asymptomatic carotid stenosis greater than 60% had a 5-year relative risk reduction (RRR) of 53% of ipsilateral stroke if carotid surgery was performed [Executive Committee for the Asymptomatic Carotid Atherosclerosis Study, 1995]. However, the absolute risk reduction (ARR) was small (5.9% in 5 years), as was the rate of ipsilateral stroke in the medically treated group (11.0% in 5 years, or 2.3% annually). Moreover, these results were achieved with a perioperative rate of complications (stroke or death) of only 2.3% [Executive Committee for the Asymptomatic Carotid Atherosclerosis Study, 1995]. Finally, the 5-year results were calculated on the basis of a 2-year follow-up and extrapolated, which reduces the reliability of the effect size [Executive Committee for the Asymptomatic Carotid Atherosclerosis Study, 1995]. Based on this trial, the number needed to treat (NNT) to avoid one ipsilateral stroke per year is 86.

A meta-analysis of 5 trials of carotid surgery for asymptomatic carotid stenosis concluded that, although surgery reduces the incidence of ipsilateral stroke, the absolute benefit of carotid surgery is small, as the rate of stroke in medically treated patients is relatively low [Benavente et al., 1998]. The authors suggested that, until high-risk subgroups have been identified, medical management remains the sensible alternative for most patients with asymptomatic carotid stenosis. Six trials were identified in the meta-analysis of the Cochrane Collaboration, but 2 were excluded on methodological grounds [Chambers et al., 2002]. Four trials with 2,203 patients were included. In 2 trials, aspirin was only given to patients in the medical group, and in 2, all patients received aspirin. The net excess 'perioperative stroke or death' rate in the surgical group was 2.7% with an RR of 6.52% (95% CI 2.66–15.96). The rates of 'perioperative stroke or death or subsequent ipsilateral stroke' were 6.8% in the medical group

Table 2. RRR, ARR and NNT to avoid 1 major vascular event per year in patients with antithrombotic therapy (modified from Hankey and Warlow [1999])

Disease	Treatment	RRR %	ARR/ year, %	NNT to avoid 1 major vascular event/year
Non-cardioembolic ischaemic stroke or TIA	ASA/placebo	13	1.0	100
	ASA + DYP/ASA	15	0.9	111
	ASA + DYP/placebo	19	1.2	53
	Clopidogrel/ASA	13	0.6	166
AF (primary prevention)	Warfarin/placebo	62	2.7	37
	ASA/placebo	22	1.5	67
AF (secondary prevention)	Warfarin/placebo	67	8	13
	ASA/placebo	21	2.5	40

ASA = Aspirin; DYP = dipyridamole.

vs. 4.9% in the surgical group (RR: 0.73; 95% CI: 0.52–1.02) favouring surgery. The rates of 'any stroke or perioperative death' were 10.4% (medical) vs. 8.1% (surgical) with RR 0.79 (95% CI 0.60–1.02). The rates of 'any stroke or death' were 23.2% (medical) vs. 20.2% (surgical) with RR 0.89 (95% CI 0.76–1.04).There were too few patients in carotid surgery vs. aspirin trials to determine whether aspirin had any confounding effect on outcome. An additional analysis, including data from a fifth small unpublished trial, slightly altered the risk ratios in favour of surgery and narrowed CIs sufficiently to achieve statistical significance for each outcome. However, inclusion of these data had no appreciable effect on the RRR or ARR.

The values of RRR, ARR and NNT to avoid 1 stroke per year in patients with asymptomatic carotid stenosis >60% are shown in table 2.

Specific Issues

1 Patients with an occlusion of the ICA contralateral to the operated carotid artery do not benefit from endarterectomy [Baker et al., 2000; Straus et al., 2002].
2 The ipsilateral stroke risk increases with the degree of the stenosis [European Carotid Surgery Trialists' Collaborative Group, 1995; Inzitari et al., 2000].
3 There are no studies investigating the benefit of carotid surgery in patients undergoing major surgery or coronary bypass.
4 A subgroup analysis of the Asymptomatic Carotid Atherosclerosis Study indicates that women have significantly lower benefit from surgery than men.
5 There are no prospective trials investigating the benefit of antiplatelet drugs in patients with asymptomatic carotid stenosis [Chambers et al., 2002].

Carotid Artery Angioplasty and Stenting for Asymptomatic Stenosis

There are no data from randomised trials about the benefit and risk of carotid angioplasty, with or without stenting, compared with endarterectomy [Roubin et al., 2001].

Recommendations

1 Carotid surgery may be indicated for some asymptomatic patients with a 60–99% stenosis of the ICA. The carotid surgery-related risk for stroke or death must be less than 3% and patients with a life expectancy of at least 5 years (or under the age of 80) may benefit from surgery (level II).
2 Carotid angioplasty, with or without stenting, is not routinely recommended for patients with asymptomatic carotid stenosis. It may be considered in the context of randomised clinical trials.

Secondary Prevention

Antiplatelet Therapy

Compared with the previously published Antiplatelet Trialist's Collaboration [Antiplatelet Trialists' Collaboration, 1994] where 145 trials were evaluated, the latest publication from the Antithrombotic Trialists's Collaboration [Antithrombotic Trialists' Collaboration, 2002] involved the meta-analysis of 287 trials with 135,000 patients in comparisons with antiplatelet therapy versus controls and 77,000 in comparisons with different antiplatelet regimens. This new effort has been coined Antithrombotic Collaboration in order to consider the effect of other drug classes such as anticoagulants. The main results were summarised as a reduction of serious vascular events (which include non-fatal MI, non-fatal stroke or vascular death) by about 25% (relative percentage). In absolute terms, the events prevented included 3.6% treated for 2 years among those with previous stroke or TIA; the absolute benefits substantially outweigh the absolute risks of major extracranial bleeding [Antithrombotic Trialists' Collaboration, 2002].

The most widely studied drug was aspirin with doses of 75–150 mg daily, which were at least as effective as higher daily doses. Recommended doses of aspirin have been shown to be effective already at a low dose. Today, doses that are low (<160 mg) are considered as effective as higher doses (160–325 mg). Studies directly comparing the effects of different doses of aspirin failed to show differences in stroke recurrence between low and medium doses [The Dutch TIA Trial Study Group, 1991] or medium and high doses [Farrell et al., 1991]. Aspirin may be effective at a daily dose of 50 mg [Diener et al., 1997]. The risk/benefit ratio of adding another antithrombotic drug to aspirin has not been fully studied. However, in stroke patients with unstable angina or non-Q wave MI, a combination of clopidogrel 75 mg and aspirin 75 mg is better than aspirin [Yusuf et al., 2001].

Clopidogrel is a thienopyridine derivative, chemically related to ticlopidine, which was superior to aspirin in stroke prevention and has only a few side-effects [Hass et al., 1989; Gent et al., 1989]. The CAPRIE study is the largest study to date that has tested clopidogrel in the setting of stroke patients. It was a randomised, double-blind study, which compared the effects of 75 mg of clopidogrel with 325 mg of aspirin once daily. The aim was to reduce a composite end point which consisted of either ischaemic stroke, MI or vascular death; 19,185 patients with a previous MI or stroke, or established peripheral artery disease were randomised. After a mean follow-up period of 1.9 years, there was a significant ARR of 0.5% and an RRR of 8.7% in favour of clopidogrel [CAPRIE Steering Committee, 1996]. Thus, clopidogrel is slightly more effective than aspirin in preventing a composite end point of vascular events. It is the agent of choice in patients with contraindications to, or adverse effects on, aspirin and may be more effective in higher-risk patients (i.e., with a previous stroke, peripheral artery disease, symptomatic CHD and DM) and after coronary surgery [Bhatt et al., 2000].

The European Stroke Prevention Study II was a randomised, double-blind, placebo-controlled trial that compared aspirin alone (50 mg daily), modified-release dipyridamole alone (200 mg twice daily), aspirin plus dipyridamole and placebo in the secondary prevention of stroke [Diener et al., 1996]: 6,602 patients that had suffered either a TIA or stroke were randomised. Fatal/non-fatal stroke, death from any cause, and stroke and/or death were assessed after a follow-up period of 2 years. The 2-year RRR of stroke in the aspirin plus dipyridamole group (37.0%) was significantly higher than in either the aspirin group (18.1%) or the dipyridamole group (16.3%). The 2-year rate of recurrent stroke was 9.5% with aspirin + dipyridamole, 12.5% with aspirin, 12.8% with dipyridamole alone and 15.2% with placebo. There was a significant difference for the comparisons aspirin + dipyridamole vs. placebo (<0.001), aspirin vs. placebo ($p = 0.013$), aspirin + dipyridamole vs. aspirin ($p = 0.006$) and dipyridamole vs. placebo (0.039). The results of the comparison between aspirin + dipyridamole versus placebo confirms the findings in the European Stroke Prevention Study [Diener et al., 1996]. The combination treatment doubles the effect of aspirin alone [Diener et al., 1996]. The results of the European Stroke Prevention Study [Diener et al., 1996] were at odds with all prior trials with dipyridamole alone or in association with aspirin, but it was also the only trial sufficiently powered to show a statistically significant difference.

Specific Issues

1. The incidence of major bleeding complications is independent of the dose of aspirin.
2. The incidence of gastro-intestinal disturbances with aspirin is dose dependent. Lower doses are safer.
3. The treatment of patients who have a recurrent vascular event on antithrombotic therapy remains unsettled. Such patients should be re-evaluated for pathophysiology and risk factors. Patients without cardiac sources of embolism who suffered a recurrent event while under aspirin did not benefit from warfarin.

Recommendations

1. Appropriate antiplatelet therapy should be given to prevent stroke recurrence and further vascular events (level I). There are three treatment options that may all be considered as first choice depending on patient characteristics.
2. Aspirin (50–325 mg) should be given to reduce stroke recurrence (level I).
3. Where available, the combination of aspirin (50 mg) and long-release dipyridamole (200 mg twice daily) can be given as first choice to reduce the risk of stoke recurrence (level I).
4. Clopidogrel is slightly more effective than aspirin in the prevention of further vascular events (level I). It may also be prescribed as first choice or when aspirin and dipyridamole are not tolerated (level IV) and in high-risk patients (level III).
5. Patients with TIA or ischaemic stroke and unstable angina or non-Q wave MI should be treated with a combination of clopidogrel 75 mg and aspirin 75 mg (level III).
6. Patients starting treatment with thienopyridine derivatives should receive clopidogrel instead of ticlopidine because it has fewer side-effects (level III).
7. In patients who cannot be treated by aspirin or thienopyridine derivatives, long-release dipyridamole alone (200 mg twice daily) may be used as an alternative (level II).

Anticoagulation

Cardioembolic Stroke

Oral anticoagulation (INR 2.0–3.0) reduces the risk of recurrent stroke in patients with non-rheumatic AF and recent ischaemic stroke [The European Atrial Fibrillation Study Group, 1995]. The risk and benefit ratio of direct thrombin antagonists is under investigation.

Oral anticoagulation therapy should also be considered for other established potential causes of cardiac embolism. Although evidence from randomised trials is lacking, long-term anticoagulation is routinely used for stroke patients with mechanical prosthetic valves. In this setting, a higher INR of between 3.0 and 4.0 is recommended [Cannegieter et al., 1995; Fuster et al., 2001]. Long-term anticoagulation with an INR of 2.0–3.0 of patients with rheumatic valvular heart disease, recent MI, heart failure, cardiomyopathy or arrhythmia other than AF should be considered.

Non-Cardioembolic Ischaemic Stroke

The Stroke Prevention in Reversible Ischaemia Trial was an open randomised study that compared the effect of 30 mg of aspirin with that of high-level anticoagulation (target INR 3.5, range 3.0–4.5) in patients with ischaemic stroke of presumed arterial origin [The Stroke Prevention in Reversible Ischemia Trial Study Group, 1997]. The trial was stopped early because of excessive mortality and major bleeding in anticoagulated patients. The Warfarin-Antiplatelet Recurrent Stroke Study (WARSS) [Mohr et al., 2001] was a double-blind, randomised clinical trial comparing aspirin (325 mg per day) with warfarin (target INR range 1.4–2.8) in 2,206 patients with a recent history of non-cardio-embolic ischaemic stroke within 30 days. No difference between aspirin and warfarin in preventing recurrent ischaemic stroke or death was found over 2 years.

Table 2 provides RRR, ARR and NNT for antithrombotic therapies in stroke prevention.

Specific Issues

1 Some retrospective studies suggest that anticoagulation may be beneficial in specific circumstances: aortic atheroma [Dressler et al., 1998], intracranial stenosis [Chimowitz et al., 1995] and basilar artery dolichoectasia [Echiverri et al., 1989]. There are no consistent data relating to anticoagulation after arterial dissection.

2 Oral anticoagulation should probably be avoided in elderly patients with leukoaraiosis [The Stroke Prevention in Reversible Ischaemia Trial Study Group, 1997].

3 It is unclear if patients with a patent foramen ovale benefit from oral anticoagulation. Patients without proven deep vein thrombosis or associated atrial septal aneurysm should probably be given aspirin. The role of anticoagulation and closure of the patent foramen ovale remains to be elucidated [Mas et al., 2001].

Recommendations

1 Oral anticoagulation (INR 2.0–3.0) is indicated after ischaemic stroke associated with AF (level I). Oral anticoagulation is not advisable in patients with comorbid conditions such as falls, epilepsy, severe dementia or gastro-intestinal bleedings.

2 Patients with prosthetic heart valves should receive long-term anticoagulation therapy with a target INR between 2.5 and 3.5 or higher (level II).

3 Patients with proven cardio-embolic stroke should be anticoagulated, if the risk of recurrence is high, with a target INR between 2. and 3.0 (level III).

4 Anticoagulation should not be used after non-cardio-embolic ischaemic stroke, except in some specific situations, such as aortic atheroma, intracranial stenosis, cervical artery dissection and basilar artery dolichoectasia (level IV).

Antihypertensive Treatment

There is good evidence that BP is a determinant of the risk of stroke among both normotensive and hypertensive individuals [Rodgers et al., 1996]. However, there has been no strong evidence until recently that reducing BP after stroke reduces the rate of new vascular events or death. A meta-analysis from 9 randomised controlled trials on antihypertensive drugs, in which a small number of stroke survivors had been included, led to an estimated RRR of 29% (95% CI 5–47) [The INDIANA Project Collaborators, 1997], but these trials suffered severe limitations.

The PATS trial assessed indapamide (2.5 mg daily, a thiazide-like diuretic) in a double-blind placebo-controlled trial involving 5,665 Chinese patients with high BP and recent stroke or TIA [PATS Collaborating Group, 1995]: indapamide lowered BP by 5/2 mm Hg and reduced the risk of recurrent stroke by 29% (ARR 2.9% over 3 years).

The HOPE study showed an effective prevention of secondary ischaemic events by an ACE inhibitor (ramipril) in stroke patients [Yusuf et al., 2000]. Although 1,013 patients with a history of stroke were included in the HOPE study, this trial cannot be considered as a secondary prevention trial after stroke: patients were eligible if they had either evidence of a vascular disease (including stroke) or DM plus another vascular risk factor, and neither heart failure nor left ventricular hypertrophy. The occurrence of the primary outcome (MI, stroke, death from cardiovascular causes) was significantly reduced in the ramipril group as compared with the placebo group (RRR: 0.78; 95% CI: 0.70–0.86). This result was observed despite a modest reduction in BP in the ramipril group and was also present in the subgroup of patients who had already had a stroke at inclusion [Bosch et al., 2002].

The Perindopril Protection against Recurrent Stroke Study (PROGRESS) was a double-blind, randomised trial comparing perindopril (4 mg daily), with or without indapamide (2–2.5 mg daily), versus placebo for the prevention of recurrent ischaemic stroke in individuals with a history of non-disabling cerebrovascular disease (minor stroke or TIA) irrespective of BP [PROGRESS Collaborative Group, 2001]. Antihypertensive treatment was initialised at least 2 weeks after stroke. The PROGRESS study included 6,105 patients and showed that lowering BP by an average of 9/4 mm Hg with a perindopril-based therapy decreased the risk of recurrent stroke by 28% versus placebo. Patients receiving both perindopril and indapamide had a mean drop in BP of 12/5 mm Hg and a 43% reduction in the risk of stroke. Interestingly, the observed benefit was achieved regardless of BP at entry and type of stroke. These beneficial effects were present in all stroke subtypes, but greater in haemorrhagic strokes (RRR: 50%; 95% CI: 33–74) and in Asians. The combination therapy prevented 1 recurrent stroke for 14 patients treated during a 5-year period.

Specific Issues

1 Although there is no convincing evidence, patients at risk of haemodynamic stroke as a consequence of occlusive or severe stenotic disease of the carotid or vertebrobasilar arteries, or who have a cardiac failure, should not have their BP lowered excessively.
2 ACE inhibitors may be considered in patients with haemodynamic brain compromise because they shift the autoregulation curve of the cerebral blood flow towards normal values.

Recommendations

1 After stroke or TIA, BP should be lowered, irrespective of its level, with a diuretic and/or an ACE inhibitor, subject to toleration of the treatment (level I).
2 The effectiveness of other classes of BP-lowering drugs has not yet been established by controlled trials.

Cholesterol-Lowering Therapy

The role of hypercholesterolaemia as a risk factor for stroke has been controversial until recently. It is now suggested that ischaemic stroke is associated with increased levels of total cholesterol, low-density lipoprotein cholesterol and triglycerides, and reduced high-density lipoprotein cholesterol levels [Iso et al., 1989; Lindenstrøm et al., 1994].

A significant reduction in stroke risk is seen in patients with a cholesterol-lowering therapy [Di Mascio et al., 2000]. However, most of this effect was driven by trials involving patients with a prior event (OR: 0.80; 95% CI: 0.71–0.91), a statin (OR: 0.77; 95% CI: 0.67–0.87) or where a reduction in total cholesterol of more than 10% was achieved (OR: 0.77; 95% CI: 0.66–0.90). Lowering cholesterol was associated with a reduction in mortality (OR: 0.85; 95% CI: 0.76–0.93) and fatal CHD (OR: 0.79; 95% CI: 0.74–0.85), but a non-significant 9% (95% CI: –13 + 37) increased risk of fatal stroke [Di Mascio et al., 2000]. A further trial found that atorvastatin reduced total stroke by 51% in patients with acute coronary syndromes [Waters et al., 2002]. One reason for discrepancies between studies may be that most studies included both ischaemic and haemorrhagic strokes, although haemorrhagic strokes have higher mortality rates and are associated with lower levels of total cholesterol [Giroud et al., 1995]. However, even if the incidence of haemorrhagic strokes was increased with statins, this risk is strongly outweighed by the significant reduction in vascular events (OR: 0.69; 95% CI: 0.59–0.80) and overall mortality (OR: 0.79; 95% CI: 0.70–0.89). Stroke incidence is reduced by a smaller degree than CHD, probably because the burden of CHD is greater in the age category in which most trials were performed. In the latest meta-analysis, 57 patients would need to be treated with statins to prevent 1 stroke per year [Straus et al., 2002].

Although there are no completed statin trial conducted in stroke patients, the MRC/BHF Heart Protection Study had a subgroup of 1,820 patients with previous stroke or TIA and without CHD [Heart Protection Study Collaborative Group, 2002]. Simvastatin (40 mg daily) reduced the risk of recurrent vascular events in this subgroup by 24%. The RR of any stroke was lowered by 25% across the whole trial involving patients with vascular disease and did not increase the risk of haemorrhagic stroke [Heart Protection Study Collaborative Group, 2002].

The beneficial effect of statins in reducing stroke in patients with vascular disease appears to be independent of other risk factors (age, gender, cholesterol level) and prophylactic measures, including treatment with aspirin, ACE inhibitors and β-RA [Plehn et al., 1999; Heart Protection Study Collaborative Group, 2002].

The PROSPER trial showed that a similar reduction in the risk of coronary events was observed under pravastatin in older individuals, without a significant effect on stroke and cognition during a mean follow-up of 3 years [Shepherd et al., 2002].

There is also evidence that fibrates can reduce the risk of stroke, as shown in the VA-HIT study of gemfibrozil [Bloomfield Rubins et al., 2001].

Data from randomised trials of any intervention aiming to decrease cholesterol levels in patients with prior stroke did not find evidence of benefit or harm [Manktelow et al., 2002]. Nevertheless, this meta-analysis did not include results from stroke patients assessed in the Heart Protection Study and the PROSPER trial.

Recommendation

1 Patients with a history of ischaemic stroke or TIA should be considered for statin (simvastatin) therapy (level I).

Hormone Replacement Therapy

Many observational studies have found a relationship between oestrogen replacement therapy and a reduced risk of vascular events in postmenopausal women [Finucane et al., 1993]. With the exception of the Framingham Heart Study, in which a 2.6-fold increase in stroke rate was observed [Wilson et al., 1995], other studies reported a slight decrease in stroke risk [Falkeborn et al., 1993; Finucane et al., 1993]. The RR of stroke among hormone replacement therapy users was 0.96 (95% CI 0.23–1.46) [Grady et al., 1992]. However, all these studies had methodological limitations [Goldstein et al., 2001]. For example, reduction of vascular events might be attributable to lifestyle differences between oestrogen users and non-users rather than to oestrogen therapy [Barrett-Connor, 1991]. Oestrogen replacement therapy may have favourable effects on lipids, thrombosis, coagulation, vascular tone, and inflammation [Viscoli et al., 2001].

The first placebo-controlled study of oestrogen replacement therapy for the secondary prevention of CHD in postmenopausal women was the Heart and Oestrogen/Progestin Replacement Study [Hulley et al., 1998]. It showed that the combination of progestin and oestrogen did not reduce the incidence of coronary events and total mortality after a 4-year period of follow-up. The Women's Oestrogen for Stroke Trial was a placebo-controlled randomised trial of oestrogen replacement therapy for the secondary prevention of ischaemic stroke [Viscoli et al., 2001]. During a mean follow-up of 2.8 years, the RR of combined stroke and death in the oestrogen group was 1.1 (95% CI 0.8–1.4); oestrogen did not reduce the risk of death alone (RR: 1.2; 95% CI: 0.8–1.8) or of non-fatal stroke (RR: 1.0; 95% CI: 0.7–1.4). The risk of fatal stroke was higher in the oestrogen group (RR: 2.9; 95% CI: 0.9–9.0) and non-fatal strokes were associated with slightly worse functional deficits [Viscoli et al., 2001]. Explanations for such results are unclear, but oestrogens may increase sensitivity to ischaemia by modulating the excitatory effects of glutamate or the inhibitory effects of GABA [Viscoli et al., 2001].

Recommendation

1 There is no indication to use hormone replacement therapy for secondary stroke prevention in postmenopausal women (level II).

Smoking

Smoking cessation leads to an early reduction in risk of both CHD (50% within 1 year; 100% by 5 years) and stroke at any age [Kawachi et al., 1993; Wannamethee et al., 1995; Wolf et al., 1988]. However, switching to pipe or cigar smoking confers little benefit, emphasising the need for complete cessation [Wells, 1994].

The population-attributable risk associated with all forms of tobacco exposure is substantial, with current smoking contributing to approximately half of strokes if we consider a population-attributable risk of 18% for current smoking, 6% for former smoking and 12% for to environmental exposure [Goldstein et al., 2001]. If all 3,600 TIA/stroke patients who smoke, in a population of 1 million people [Hankey and Warlow, 1999], stopped smoking, the annual number of strokes might be reduced from 252 (7%) to 168 (4.7%), avoiding about 84 (3.5%) of 2,400 strokes. Forty-three smokers need to stop smoking to avoid 1 stroke [Hankey and Warlow, 1999]. The data on smoking cessation are available only from observational studies. Table 3 provides RRR, ARR and NNT for risk factor modifications in stroke prevention.

Recommendation

1 All smokers should stop smoking, especially the patients who had stroke (level IV).

Carotid Surgery

Although carotid surgery has been performed since the 1950s, it was only in the 1990s that the results of large randomised clinical trials clarified the indications for surgery [Biller et al., 1998]. The NASCET [North American Symptomatic Carotid Endarterectomy Trial Collaborators, 1991] and ECST [European Carotid Surgery Trialists' Collaborative Group, 1991] reported that surgery was efficacious for symptomatic patients with ipsilateral carotid stenosis greater than 70%. Although these trials

Table 3. RRR, ARR and NNT to avoid 1 major vascular event per year in patients with risk factors modification (modified from Hankey and Warlow [1999])

Clinical condition	Treatment	RRR %	ARR %	NNT to avoid 1 stroke/year
General population with increased BP	antihypertensive	42	0.2	94
Post-stroke/TIA with increased BP	antihypertensive	31	2.2	45
Post-stroke/TIA with normal BP	antihypertensive	28	4	42
Post-stroke/TIA	statins	24	1.7	59
	smoking cessation	33	2.3	43

used different methods to measure stenosis, it is possible to convert the percentage of stenosis from one method to another and there is little difference in their ability to predict ipsilateral stroke [Rothwell et al., 1994].

In the NASCET, patients who underwent carotid surgery had an absolute reduction of 17% in the risk of ipsilateral stroke at 2 years (RRR of 65%) [North American Symptomatic Carotid Endarterectomy Trial Collaborators, 1991]. The study showed that the NNT was 6 patients to prevent 1 stroke. However, these results were achieved with a perioperative morbidity and mortality of 5.5% (all strokes and deaths) [North American Symptomatic Carotid Endarterectomy Trial Collaborators, 1991]. Restricting the analysis to major stroke and death resulted in a rate of 2.1%. These rates did not include a risk of complication of angiography of about 1% [North American Symptomatic Carotid Endarterectomy Trial Collaborators, 1991]. The authors therefore warn that, if perioperative complications exceed 2.1%, the benefit of carotid surgery will diminish and, if the complication rate approaches 10%, the benefit will vanish entirely.

Although the rate of perioperative complications in the ECST was higher (7.5% for death, disabling stroke or any stroke producing symptoms for more than 7 days), surgery-allocated patients still had a significant ARR of 6.5% in ipsilateral stroke and an RRR of 39% [European Carotid Surgery Trialists' Collaborative Group, 1991].

The NASCET analysis of surgery for symptomatic patients with less than 70% stenosis revealed an ARR of 6.5% and an RRR of 29% for patients with 50–69% stenosis allocated for surgery [Barnett et al., 1998]. Fifteen patients would need to be treated by carotid surgery to prevent 1 ipsilateral stroke at 5 years. The overall significance of carotid surgery in preventing ipsilateral stroke was marginal ($p = 0.045$) and the CIs overlapped in the survival curves. Logistic regression analysis identified seven characteristics that doubled the perioperative risk of stroke or death. Among these are contralateral carotid occlusion, left-sided carotid disease, less than 650 mg of aspirin per day, the absence of a history of MI or angina, an asymptomatic lesion present ipsilaterally to the stenosed artery, a history of DM and a diastolic BP higher than 90 mm Hg. The authors concluded that all risk factors should be evaluated when patients with a 50–69% stenosis are being considered for surgery.

Table 4. RRR, ARR and NNT to avoid 1 stroke per year in patients who undergo surgery for ICA stenosis (modified from Hankey and Warlow [1999])

Disease	RRR, %	ARR/ year, %	NNT to avoid 1 stroke/year
Asymptomatic (60–99%)	53	1.2	85
Symptomatic (70–99%)	65	3.8	27
Symptomatic (50–69%)	29	1.3	75
Symptomatic (<50%)	no benefit	no benefit	no benefit

According to the most recent meta-analysis of pooled data from 3 trials (ECST, NASCET and Veterans Affairs Trial 309), carotid surgery is highly beneficial for patients with a 70% symptomatic stenosis or greater, but without near-occlusion [Rothwell et al., 2003]. In the same meta-analysis, modest benefit from surgery was found in patients with a 50–69% stenosis [Rothwell et al., 2003].

In the above trials, stenosis was evaluated by angiography. Although the use of ultrasonography as a prelude to surgery is questioned [Barnett et al., 1995], it may be reasonable to proceed with carotid surgery if one or more of the following investigations show a severe stenosis: ultrasonography, magnetic resonance angiography and/or CT angiography.

Table 4 provides RRR, ARR and NNT for carotid surgery in stroke prevention.

Specific Issues

1 Elderly patients (>75 years) without organ failure or serious cardiac dysfunction benefit from carotid surgery.

2 Women with severe stenosis (>70%) should undergo carotid surgery. Women with moderate stenosis should be treated medically.
3 Patients with few risk factors who present with amaurosis fugax are only better off with medical treatment. Patients with a severe stenosis and a high-risk profile should be considered for carotid surgery.
4 Patients with mild to moderate intracranial stenosis and severe extracranial stenosis are ideal candidates for carotid surgery.
5 The benefit from carotid surgery is lower for patients with lacunar stroke.
6 Patients with leukoaraiosis should be made aware of the increased operative risk.
7 Occlusion of the contralateral ICA is not a contraindication to carotid surgery, but it carries a higher perioperative risk.
8 Continuation of aspirin is required until surgery, but heparin may be used in very severe stenosis.
9 The benefit from endarterectomy is marginal in patients with carotid near-occlusion.

Recommendations

1 Conventional angiography (level I), or one (or ideally more) of the following non-invasive investigations – duplex ultrasonography, magnetic resonance angiography or CT angiography (level III) – may be used to identify and quantify carotid artery stenosis.
2 Carotid surgery is indicated for patients with stenosis of 70–99% without a severe neurological deficit with recent (<180 days) ischaemic events. This is valid only for centres with a perioperative complication rate (all strokes and death) of less than 6% (level I).
3 Carotid surgery may be indicated for certain patients with stenosis of 50–69% without a severe neurological deficit. This is valid only for centres with a perioperative complication rate (all strokes and death) of less than 6%. The subgroup of patients most likely to benefit from surgery is males with recent hemispheric symptoms (level III).
4 Carotid surgery is not recommended for patients with stenosis of less than 50% (level I).
5 Carotid surgery should not be performed in centres not exhibiting low complication rates similar to those seen in NASCET or ECST (level I).
6 Patients should remain on antithrombotic therapy before, during and after surgery (level II).
7 Patients should be followed up by the referring physician as well as the surgeon (level IV).

Extracranial-Intracranial Anastomosis (EC-IC Bypass)

A large randomised trial involving 1,377 patients showed that anastomosis between the superficial temporal and middle cerebral arteries was not beneficial in preventing stroke in patients with middle cerebral artery or ICA stenosis or occlusion [The EC/IC Bypass Study Group, 1985]. Further studies are necessary to determine whether a subgroup of patients would benefit from carotid artery bypass, and the ongoing COSS trial is aimed to answer this question [Mitka, 2002].

Carotid Angioplasty and Stenting

Percutaneous transluminal angioplasty (PTA) is a potentially valuable technique. Its advantages over carotid surgery are short hospital stays, the avoidance of general anaesthesia and surgical incision and the ability to treat surgically inaccessible sites, such as the high cervical ICA [CAVATAS Investigators, 2001]. Moreover, carotid PTA and stenting may be the most effective means of treating restenosis after initial carotid surgery [Yadav et al., 1996]. Results from a large series of patients treated with PTA, with or without stents, suggest that the procedural rate of complications is comparable with that of carotid surgery [Gil-Peralta et al., 1996]. In the future, carotid angioplasty and stenting may be good alternatives for carotid surgery but that time has not yet arrived. Angioplasty was compared with carotid surgery in the Carotid and Vertebral Artery Transluminal Angioplasty Study (CAVATAS), a randomised clinical trial [CAVATAS Investigators, 2001]. The 30-day death and stroke rate of carotid surgery was 9.9% and that of angioplasty 10.0% in the CAVATAS, i.e. both therapies carried a higher risk than in NASCET, ECST or ACAS [CAVATAS Investigators, 2001]. Since the beginning of CAVATAS, new techniques such as cerebral protection by an umbrella or occlusive balloon distal to the site of angioplasty and combining angioplasty with stenting to decrease the risks of dissection and restenosis have become available. For these reasons, we are waiting for the results of ongoing trials. The use of carotid angioplasty and stenting should be limited to well-designed, well-conducted, randomised studies with careful dispassionate overview according to the statement of the American Heart Association Expert Group [Bettmann et al., 1998] or to patients with symptomatic stenoses and contraindications to carotid surgery or with stenosis at surgically inaccessible sites, re-stenosis after initial carotid surgery or stenosis following radiation. Patients should receive a combination of clopidogrel and aspirin immediately before, during and at least 1 month after stenting [Bertrand et al., 2000].

Recommendations

1 Carotid PTA may be performed for patients with contraindications to carotid surgery or with stenosis at surgically inaccessible sites (level IV).
2 Carotid PTA and stenting may be indicated for patients with restenosis after initial carotid surgery or stenosis following radiation (level IV).
3 Patients should receive a combination of clopidogrel and aspirin immediately before, during and at least 1 month after stenting (level IV).

References

Abbott R, Yin Y, Reed D, Yano K: Risk of stroke in male cigarette smokers. N Engl J Med 1986; 315:717–720.

Adams HP Jr, Brott TG, Crowell RM, Furlan AJ, Gomez CR, Grotta J, Helgason CM, Marler JR, Woolson RF, Zivin JA, et al: Guidelines for the management of patients with acute ischaemic stroke. A statement for healthcare professionals from a special writing group of the Stroke Council, American Heart Association. Stroke 1994;25;1901–1914.

Antiplatelet Trialists' Collaboration. Collaborative overview of randomised trials of antiplatelet therapy. 1. Prevention of death, myocardial infarction, and stroke by prolonged antiplatelet therapy in various categories of patients. BMJ 1994;308:81–106.

Antithrombotic Trialists' Collaboration: Collaborative meta-analysis of randomized trials of antiplatelet therapy for prevention of death, myocardial infarction, and stroke in high risk patients. BMJ 2002;324:71–86.

Baker WH, Howard VJ, Howard G, Toole JF, for the ACAS Investigators: Effect of contralateral occlusion on long-term efficacy of endarterectomy in the Asymptomatic Carotid Atherosclerosis Study (ACAS). Stroke 2000;31:2330–2334.

Barnett H, Eliasziw M, Meldrum H: Drugs and surgery in the prevention of ischemic stroke. N Engl J Med 1995;332:238–248.

Barnett HJ, Taylor DW, Eliasziw M, Fox AJ, Ferguson GG, Haynes RB, Rankin RN, Clagett GP, Hachinski VC, Sackett DL, Thorpe KE, Meldrum HE: Benefit of endarterectomy in patients with symptomatic moderate or severe stenosis. N Engl J Med 1998;339:1415–1425.

Barrett-Connor E: Postmenopausal oestrogen and prevention bias. Ann Intern Med 1991;115: 455–456.

Benavente O, Moher D, Pham B: Carotid endarterectomy for asymptomatic carotid stenosis: A meta-analysis. BMJ 1998;317:1477–1480.

Bertrand ME, Rupprecht HJ, Urban P, Gershlick AH: Double-blind study of the safety of clopidogrel with and without a loading dose in combination with aspirin compared with ticlopidine in combination with aspirin after coronary stenting: The clopidogrel aspirin stent international cooperative study (CLASSICS). Circulation 2000;102:624–629.

Bettmann MA, Katzen BT, Whisnant J, et al: Carotid stenting and angioplasty. A statement for healthcare professionals from the councils on cardiovascular radiology, Stroke, cardio-thoracic and vascular surgery, epidemiology and prevention, and clinical cardiology, American Heart Association. Stroke 1998;29:336–348.

Bhatt DL, Kapadia SR, Yadav JS, Topol EJ: Update on clinical trials of antiplatelet therapy for cerebrovascular diseases. Cerebrovasc Dis 2000;10(suppl 5):34–40.

Biller J, Feinberg W, Castaldo J, Whittemore A, Harbaugh R, Dempsey R, Caplan L, et al: Guidelines for carotid endarterectomy. A statement for healthcare professionals from a special writing group of the Stroke Council, American Heart Association. Stroke 1998;97:501–509.

Bloomfield Rubins H, Davenport J, Babikian V, Brass LM, Collins D, Wexler L, Wagner S, Papademetriou V, Rutan G, Robins SJ: Reduction in stroke with gemfibrozil in men with coronary heart disease and low HDL cholesterol: The Veterans Affairs HDL Intervention Trial (VA-HIT). Circulation 2001;103:2828–2833.

Bosch J, Yusuf S, Pogue J, Sleight P, Lonn E, Rangoonwala B, Davies R, Ostergren J, Probstfield J, and the HOPE Investigators: Use of ramipril in preventing stroke: Double-blind randomised trial. BMJ 2002;324;699–702.

Bronner L, Kanter D, Manson J: Primary prevention of stroke. N Engl J Med 1995;333: 1392–1400.

Cannegieter S, Rosendaal F, Witzen A, Van Der Meer F, Vandenbroucke J, Briët E: Optimal oral anticoagulation therapy in patients with mechanical heart valves. N Engl J Med 1995; 333:11–17.

CAPRIE Steering Committee: A randomised, blinded trial of clopidogrel versus aspirin in patients at risk of ischaemic events (CAPRIE). Lancet 1996;348:1329–1339.

CAVATAS Investigators: Endovascular versus surgical treatment in patients with carotid stenosis in the Carotid and Vertebral Artery Transluminal Angioplasty Study: A randomised trial. Lancet 2001;357:1729–1737.

Chambers BR, You RX, Donnan GA: Carotid endarterectomy for asymptomatic carotid stenosis (Cochrane review); in: Cochrane Library, Issue 4, 2002. Update Software.

Chimowitz MI, Kokkinos J, Strong J, Brown MB, Levine SR, Silliman S, Pessin MS, Weichel E, Sila CA, Furlan AJ: The Warfarin-Aspirin Symptomatic Intracranial Disease Study. Neurology 1995;45:1488–1493.

Colditz GA, Bonita R, Stampfer MJ, Willett WC, Rosner B, Speizer FE, Hennekens CH: Cigarette smoking and risk of stroke in middle-aged women. N Engl J Med 1988;318:937–941.

Connolly SJ, Laupacis A, Gent M, Roberts RS, Cairns JA, Joyner C: Canadian Atrial Fibrillation Anticoagulation (CAFA) Study. J Am Coll Cardiol 1991;18:349–355.

Côté R, Battista RN, Abrahamowicz M, Langlois Y, Bourque F, Mackey A: Lack of effect of aspirin in asymptomatic patients with carotid bruit and substantial carotid narrowing. Ann Intern Med 1995;123:649–655.

Dahlof B, Devereux RB, Kjeldsen SE, Julius S, Beevers G, Faire U, Fyhrquist F, Ibsen H, Kristiansson K, Lederballe-Pedersen O, Lindholm LH, Nieminen MS, Omvik P, Oparil S, Wedel H: Cardiovascular morbidity and mortality in the Losartan Intervention for Endpoint reduction in hypertension study (LIFE): A randomised trial against atenolol. Lancet 2002;359: 995–1003.

Diener HC, Cunha L, Forbes C, Sivenius J, Smets P, Lowenthal A: European Stroke Prevention Study. 2. Dipyridamole and acetylsalicylic acid in the secondary prevention of stroke. J Neurol Sci 1996;143:1–13.

Donahue RP, Abbott RD. Alcohol and haemorrhagic stroke. Lancet 1986;ii:515–516.

Downs JR, Clearfield M, Weis S, Whitney E, Shapiro DR, Beere PA, Langendorfer A, Stein EA, Kruyer W, Gotto AM Jr: Primary prevention of acute coronary events with lovastatin in men and women with average cholesterol levels: Results of AFCAPS/TexCAPS. Air Force/Texas Coronary Atherosclerosis Prevention Study. JAMA 1998;279:1615–1622.

Dressler FA, Craig WR, Castello R, Labovitz AJ: Mobile aortic atheroma and systemic emboli: Efficacy of anticoagulation and influence of plaque morphology on recurrent stroke. J Am Coll Cardiol 1998;31:134–138.

Eastern Stroke and Coronary Heart Disease Collaborative Research Group: Blood pressure, cholesterol, and stroke in eastern Asia. Lancet 1988;352:1801–1807.

Echiverri HC, Rubino FA, Gupta SR, Gujrati M: Fusiform aneurysm of the vertebrobasilar arterial system. Stroke 1989;20:1741–1747.

ETDRS Investigators: Aspirin effects on mortality and morbidity in patients with diabetes mellitus. Early Treatment Diabetic Retinopathy Study report 14. JAMA 1992;268:1292–1300.

European Carotid Surgery Trialists' Collaborative Group: MRC European Carotid Surgery Trial: Interim results for symptomatic patients with severe (70–99%) or with mild (0–29%) carotid stenosis. Lancet 1991;337:1235–1243.

European Carotid Surgery Trialists Collaborative Group: Risk of stroke in the distribution of an asymptomatic carotid artery. Lancet 1995;345: 209–212.

Executive Committee for the Asymptomatic Carotid Atherosclerosis Study: Endarterectomy for asymptomatic carotid artery stenosis. JAMA 1995;273:1421–1428.

Ezekowitz MD, Bridgers SL, James KE, et al: Warfarin in the prevention of stroke associated with nonrheumatic atrial fibrillation. N Engl J Med 1992;327:1406–1412.

Falkeborn M, Persson I, Terent A, et al: Hormone replacement therapy and the risk of stroke: Follow-up of a population-based cohort in Sweden. Arch Intern Med 1993;153:1201–1209.

Farrell B, Godwin J, Richards S, Warlow C: The United Kingdom transient ischaemic attack (UK-TIA) aspirin trial: Final results. J Neurol Neurosurg Psychiatry 1991;54:1044–1054.

Fine-Edelstein JS, Wolf PA, O'Leary DH, Poehlman H, Belanger AJ, Kase CS, D'Agostino RB: Precursors of extracranial carotid atherosclerosis in the Framingham study. Neurology 1994; 44:1046–1050.

Finucane FF, Madans JH, Bush TL, Wolf PH, Kleinman JC: Decreased risk of stroke among postmenopausal hormone users. Arch Intern Med 1993;153:73–79.
Fuster V, Ryden LE, Asinger RW, Cannom DS, Crijns HJ, Frye RL, Halperin JL, Kay GN, Klein WW, Levy S, McNamara RL, Prystowsky EN, Wann LS, Wyse DG, Gibbons RJ, Antman EM, Alpert JS, Faxon DP, Fuster V, Gregoratos G, Hiratzka LF, Jacobs AK, Russell RO, Smith SC, Klein WW, Alonso-Garcia A, Blomstrom-Lundqvist C, De Backer G, Flather M, Hradec J, Oto A, Parkhomenko A, Silber S, Torbicki A: ACC/AHA/ESC guidelines for the management of patients with atrial fibrillation: Executive summary. A report of the American College of Cardiology/American Heart Association Task Force on Practice Guidelines and the European Society of Cardiology Committee for Practice Guidelines and Policy Conferences (Committee to Develop Guidelines for the Management of Patients with Atrial Fibrillation): Developed in Collaboration with the North American Society of Pacing and Electrophysiology. J Am Coll Cardiol 2001;38:1231–1266.
de Gaetano G: Low-dose aspirin and vitamin E in people at cardiovascular risk: A randomised trial in general practice. Collaborative Group of the Primary Prevention Project. Lancet 2001;357:89–95.
Gent M, Blakely JA, Easton JD, Ellis DJ, Hachinski VC, Harbison JW, Panak E, Roberts RS, Sicurella J, Turpie AG: The Canadian-American Ticlopidine Study (CATS) in thromboembolic stroke. Lancet 1989;i:1215–1220.
Gil-Peralta A, Mayol A, Marcos JR, Gonzalez A, Ruano J, Boza F, Duran F: Percutaneous transluminal angioplasty of the symptomatic atherosclerotic carotid arteries. Results, complications, and follow-up. Stroke 1996;27:2271–2273.
Giroud M, Creisson E, Fayolle H, Andre N, Becker F, Martin D, Dumas R: Risk factors for primary cerebral hemorrhage: A population-based study – The Stroke Registry of Dijon. Neuroepidemiology 1995;14:20–26.
Goldstein LB, Adams R, Becker K, et al: Primary prevention of ischemic stroke: A statement for healthcare professionals from the stroke council of the American Heart Association. Circulation 2001;103:163–182.
Grady D, Herrington D, Bittner V, Blumenthal R, Davidson M, Hlatky M, Hsia J, Hulley S, Herd A, Khan S, Newby LK, Waters D, Vittinghoff E, Wenger N: Cardiovascular disease outcomes during 6.8 years of hormone therapy: Heart and Estrogen/Progestin Replacement Study follow-up (HERS II). JAMA 2002;288:49–57.
Grady D, Rubin SM, Petitti DB, et al: Hormone therapy to prevent disease and prolong life in postmenopausal women. Ann Intern Med 1992;117:1016–1037.
Grodstein F, Manson JE, Stampfer MJ: Postmenopausal hormone use and secondary prevention of coronary events in the nurses' health study. A prospective, observational study. Ann Intern Med 2001;135:1–8.
Hankey GJ, Warlow CP: Treatment and secondary prevention of stroke: Evidence, costs, and effects on individuals and populations. Lancet 1999;354:1457–1463.
Hansson L, Zanchetti A, Carruthers S, Dahlof B, Elmfeldt D, Julius S, Menard J, Rahn KH, Wedel H, Westerling S: Effects of intensive blood-pressure lowering and low-dose aspirin in patients with hypertension: Principal results of the Hypertension Optimal Treatment (HOT) randomised trial. Lancet 1998;351: 1755–1762.
Hart RG, Halperin JL, McBride R, Benavente O, Man-Son-Hing M, Kronmal RA: Aspirin for the primary prevention of stroke and other major vascular events: Meta-analysis and hypotheses. Arch Neurol 2000a;57:326–332.
Hart RG, Pearce LA, Rothbart RM, McAnulty JH, Asinger RW, Halperin JL: Stroke with intermittent atrial fibrillation: Incidence and predictors during aspirin therapy. Stroke Prevention in Atrial Fibrillation Investigators. J Am Coll Cardiol 2000b;35:183–187.
Hart RG, Sherman DG, Easton JD, Cairns J: Prevention of stroke in patients with nonvalvular atrial fibrillation. Neurology 1998;51:674–681.
Hass WK, Easton JD, Adams HP Jr, Pryse-Phillips W, Molony BA, Anderson S, Kamm B: A randomised trial comparing ticlopidine hydrochloride with aspirin for the prevention of stroke in high-risk patients. N Engl J Med 1989;321;501–507.
He K, Rimm EB, Merchant A, Rosner BA, Stampfer MJ, Willett WC, Ascherio A: Fish consumption and risk of stroke in men. JAMA 2002; 288:3130–3136.
Heart Protection Study Collaborative Group: MRC/BHF Heart Protection Study of cholesterol lowering with simvastatin in 20,536 high-risk individuals: A randomised placebo-controlled trial. Lancet 2002;360:7–22.
Hebert PR, Gaziano JM, Hennekens CH: An overview of trials of cholesterol lowering and risk of stroke. Arch Intern Med 1995;155:50–55.
Hu FB, Willett WC: Optimal diets for prevention of coronary heart disease. JAMA 2002;288: 2569–2578.
Hulley S, Grady D, Bush T, Furberg C, Herrington D, Riggs B, Vittinghoff E: Randomised trial of estrogen plus progestin for secondary prevention of coronary heart disease in postmenopausal women. Heart and Estrogen/Progestin Replacement Study (HERS) Research Group. JAMA 1998;280:605–613.
Inzitari D, Eliasziw M, Gates P, Sharpe BL, Chan RKT, Meldrum HE, Barnett HJM: The causes and risk of stroke in patients with asymptomatic internal-carotid-artery stenosis. N Engl J Med 2000;342:1693–1700.
Iso H, Jacobs DR Jr, Wentworth D, et al: Serum cholesterol levels and six-year mortality from stroke in 350,977 men screened for the multiple risk factor intervention trial. N Engl J Med 1989;320:904–910.
Kawachi I, Colditz GA, Stampfer MJ, WC, Manson JE, Rosner B, Speizer FE, Hennekens CH: Smoking cessation and decreased risk of stroke in women. JAMA 1993;269:232–236.
Laupacis A, Albers G, Dalen J, Dunn M, Jacobson A, Singer D: Antithrombotic therapy in atrial fibrillation. Chest 1998;114:579–589.
Lee IM, Hennekens CH, Berger K, Buring JE, Manson JE: Exercise and risk of stroke in male physicians. Stroke 1999;30:1–6.
Lindenstrøm E, Boysen G, Nyboe J: Influence of total cholesterol, high density lipoprotein cholesterol, and triglycerides on risk of cerebrovascular disease: The Copenhagen City Heart Study. BMJ 1994;309:11–15.
Lip G, Lowe G: ABC of atrial fibrillation. Antithrombotic treatment for atrial fibrillation. BMJ 1996;312:45–49.
Manktelow B, Gillies C, Potter JF: Interventions in the management of serum lipids for preventing stroke recurrence. Cochrane Database Syst Rev 2002;(3):CD002091.
Di Mascio R, Marchili R, Tognoni G: Cholesterol reduction and stroke occurrence: An overview of randomized clinical trials. Cerebrovascular Dis 2000;10:85–92.
Mas JL, Arquizan C, Lamy C, Zuber M, Cabanes L, Derumeaux G, Coste J: Recurrent cerebrovascular events associated with patent foramen ovale, atrial sptal aneurysm, or both. N Engl J Med 2001;345:1740–1746.
Meade T: Low dose warfarin and aspirin in preventing IHD. Practitioner 1998;242:799–803.
Mitka M: PET theory applied to stroke prevention. JAMA 2002;288:2531.
Mohr JP, Thompson JL, Lazar RM, Levin B, Sacco RL, Furie KL, Kistler JP, Albers GW, Pettigrew LC, Adams HP Jr, Jackson CM, Pullicino P: A comparison of warfarin and aspirin for the prevention of recurrent ischemic stroke. N Engl J Med 2001;345:1444–1451.
Nadareishvili Z, Rothwell P, Beletsky V, Pagniello A, Norris J: Long-term risk of stroke and other vascular events in patients with asymptomatic carotid artery stenosis. Arch Neurol 2002;59: 1162–1166.
National Center for Health Statistics: Healthy People 2000 Review, 1989–1999. Hyattsville, US Dept of Health and Human Services, 1999.
Neal B, MacMahon S, Chapman N: Effects of ACE inhibitors, calcium antagonists, and other blood-pressure-lowering drugs: Results of prospectively designed overviews of randomised trials. Blood Pressure Lowering Treatment Trialists' Collaboration. Lancet 2000;356: 1955–1964.
Norris JW, Zhu CZ, Bornstein NM, Chambers BR: Vascular risks of asymptomatic carotid stenosis. Stroke 1991;22:1485–1490.
North American Symptomatic Carotid Endarterectomy Trial Collaborators. Beneficial effect of carotid endarterectomy in symptomatic patients with high-grade carotid stenosis. N Engl J Med 1991;325; 445–453.
PATS Collaborating Group: Post-stroke antihypertensive treatment study. A preliminary result. Chin Med J 1995;108:710–717.
Petersen P, Boysen G, Godtfredsen J, Andersen ED, Andersen B: Placebo-controlled, randomised trial of warfarin and aspirin for prevention of thromboembolic complications in chronic atrial fibrillation: The Copenhagen AFASAK Study. Lancet 1989;333:175–179.

Peto R, Gray R, Collins R, Wheatley K, Hennekens C, Jamrozik K, Warlow C, Hafner B, Thompson E, Norton S: Randomised trial of prophylactic daily aspirin in British male doctors. BMJ 1988;296:313–316.

Plehn JF, Davis BR, Sacks FM, Rouleau JL, Pfeffer MA, Bernstein V, Cuddy TE, Moye LA, Piller LB, Rutherford J, Simpson LM, Braunwald E: Reduction of stroke incidence after myocardial infarction with pravastatin: The Cholesterol and Recurrent Events (CARE) Study. The Care Investigators. Circulation 1999;99:216–223.

PROGRESS Collaborative Group: Randomised trial of a perindopril-based blood-pressure-lowering regimen among 6,105 individuals with previous stroke or transient ischaemic attack. Lancet 2001;358:1033–1041.

Prospective Studies Collaboration: Age-specific relevance of usual blood pressure to vascular mortality: A meta-analysis of individual data for one million adults in 61 prospective studies. Lancet 2002;360:1903–1913.

Prospective Studies Collaboration: Cholesterol, diastolic blood pressure, and stroke; 13,000 strokes in 450,000 people in 45 prospective cohorts. Lancet 1995;346:1647–1653.

Reynolds K, Lewis LB, Nolen JDL, Kinney GL, Sathya B, He J: Alcohol consumption and risk of stroke. A meta-analysis. JAMA 2003;289:579–588.

Robbins AS, Manson JE, Lee I-M, et al: Cigarette smoking and stroke in a cohort of US male physicians. Ann Intern Med 1994;120:458–462.

Rodgers A, MacMahon S, Gamble G, Slattery J, Sandercock P, Warlow C: Blood pressure and risk of stroke in patients with cerebrovascular disease. The United Kingdom Transient Ischaemic Attack Collaborative Group. BMJ 1996;313:147.

Rothwell PM, Eliasziv M, Gutnikov SA, Fox AJ, Taylor DW, Mayberg MR, Warlow CP, Barnett HJM: Analysis of pooled data from the randomized controlled trials of endarterectomy for symptomatic carotid stenosis. Lancet 2003;361;107–116.

Rothwell PM, Gibson RJ, Slattery J, Warlow CP: Prognostic value and reproducibility of measurements of carotid stenosis. A comparison of three methods on 1,001 angiograms. European Carotid Surgery Trialists' Collaborative Group. Stroke 1994;25:2440–2444.

Roubin GS, New G, Iyer SS, Vitek JJ, Al-Mubarak N, Liu MW, Yadav J, Gomez C, Kuntz RE: Immediate and late clinical outcomes of carotid artery stenting in patients with symptomatic and asymptomatic carotid artery stenosis: A 5-year prospective analysis. Circulation 2001;103:532–537.

Sacco RL: Extracranial carotid stenosis. N Engl J Med 2001;345:1113–1118.

Shepherd J, Blauw GJ, Murphy MB, Bollen EL, Buckley BM, Cobbe SM, Ford I, Gaw A, Hyland M, Jukema JW, Kamper AM, Macfarlane PW, Meinders AE, Norrie J, Packard CJ, Perry IJ, Stott DJ, Sweeney BJ, Twomey C, Westendorp RG, for the PROSPER (PROspective Study of Pravastatin in the Elderly at Risk) Study Group: Pravastatin in elderly individuals at risk of vascular disease (PROSPER): A randomised controlled trial. Lancet 2002;360:1623–1630.

Shinton R, Beevers G: Meta-analysis of relation between cigarette smoking and stroke. BMJ 1989;298:789–794.

SPAF III Writing Committee for the Stroke Prevention in Atrial Fibrillation Investigators: Patients with nonvalvular atrial fibrillation at low risk of stroke during treatment with aspirin: Stroke prevention in atrial fibrillation III study. JAMA 1998;279:1273–1277.

Staessen JA, Wang JG, Thijs L: Cardiovascular protection and blood pressure reduction: A meta-analysis. Lancet 2001;358:1305–1315.

Steering Committee of the Physicians' Health Study Research Group. Final report of the ongoing physicians health study. N Engl J Med 1989;321:129–135.

Straus SE, Majumdar SR, McAlister FA: New evidence for stroke prevention: Scientific review. JAMA 2002;288:1388–1395.

Stroke Prevention in Atrial Fibrillation Investigators: Warfarin versus aspirin for prevention of thromboembolism in atrial fibrillation: Stroke prevention in atrial fibrillation II study. Lancet 1994;343:687–691.

Suh I, Jee SH, Kim HC, Nam CM, Kim IS, Appel LJ: Low serum cholesterol and haemorrhagic stroke in men: Korea Medical Insurance Corporation Study. Lancet 2001;357:922–925.

The ALLHAT Officers and Coordinators for the ALLHAT Collaborative Research Group: Major outcomes in moderately hypercholesterolaemic, hypertensive patients randomized to pravastatin vs usual care: The Antihypertensive and Lipid-Lowering Treatment to Prevent Heart Attack Trial (ALLHAT-LLT). JAMA 2002;288:2998–3007.

The ALLHAT Officers and Coordinators for the ALLHAT Collaborative Research Group. Major cardiovascular events in hypertensive patients randomized to doxazosin versus chlorthalidone. The antihypertensive and lipid-lowering treatment to prevent heart attack trial (ALLHAT). JAMA 2000;283:1967–1975.

The Boston Area Anticoagulation Trial for Atrial Fibrillation Investigators. The effects of low-dose warfarin on the risk of stroke in patients with nonrheumatic atrial fibrillation. N Engl J Med 1990;323:1505–1511.

The Dutch TIA Trial Study Group: A comparison of two doses of aspirin (30 mg vs 283 mg a day) in patients after a transient ischaemic attack or minor ischaemic stroke. N Engl J Med 1991;325:1261–1266.

The EC/IC Bypass Study Group: Failure of extracranial-intracranial arterial bypass to reduce the risk of ischaemic stroke. Results of an international randomised trial. N Engl J Med 1985;313:1191–2000.

The European Atrial Fibrillation Study Group: Optimal oral anticoagulation therapy with nonrheumatic atrial fibrillation and recent cerebral ischemia N Engl J Med 1995;333:5–10.

The INDIANA (Individual Data Analysis of Antihypertensive Intervention Trials) Project Collaborators: Effect of antihypertensive treatment in patients having already suffered from stroke: Gathering the evidence. Stroke 1997;28:2557–2562.

The Stroke Prevention in Atrial Fibrillation Investigators: Predictors of thromboembolism in atrial fibrillation. 1. Clinical features of patients at risk. Ann Intern Med 1992;116:1–5.

The Stroke Prevention in Reversible Ischaemia Trial Study Group: A randomised trial of anticoagulants versus aspirin after cerebral ischemia of presumed arterial origin. Ann Neurol 1997;42:857–865.

Turner RC, Cull CA, Frighi V, Holman RR: Glycemic control with diet, sulfonylurea, metformin, or insulin in patients with type 2 diabetes mellitus: progressive requirement for multiple therapies (UKPDS 49). UK Prospective Diabetes Study (UKPDS) Group. JAMA 1999;281:2005–2012.

Viscoli CM, Brass LM, Kernan WN, Sarrel PM, Suissa S, Horwitz RI: A clinical trial of replacement-replacement therapy after ischemic stroke. N Engl J Med 2001;345:1243–1249.

Wannamethee SG, Shaper AG, Whincup PH, Walker M: Smoking cessation and the risk of stroke in middle-aged men. JAMA 1995;274:155–160.

Waters DD, Schwartz GG, Olsson AG, Zeiher A, Oliver MF, Ganz P, Ezekowitz M, Chaitman BR, Leslie SJ, Stern T: Effects of atorvastatin on stroke in patients with unstable angina or non-Q-wave myocardial infarction: A Myocardial Ischaemia Reduction with Aggressive Cholesterol Lowering (MIRACL) substudy. Circulation 2002;106:1690–1695.

Wells AJ: Passive smoking as a cause of heart disease. J Am Coll Cardiol 1994;24:546–554.

West of Scotland Coronary Prevention Study Group: Influence of pravastatin and plasma lipids on clinical events in the West of Scotland Coronary Prevention Study. Circulation 1998;97:1440–1445.

Wilson PW, Garrison RJ, Castelli WP: Postmenopausal oestrogen use, cigarette smoking, and cardiovascular morbidity in women over 50: The Framingham Study. N Engl J Med 1985;313:1038–1043.

Wolf Pa, D'Agostino Rb, Belanger Aj, Kannel WB: Probability of stroke: A risk profile from the Framingham Study. Stroke 1991;22:312–318.

Wolf PA, D'Agostino RB, Kannel WB, Bonita R, Belanger AJ: Cigarette smoking as a risk factor for stroke: The Framingham study. JAMA 1988;259:1025–1029.

Yadav JS, Roubin GS, King P, Iyer S, Vitek J: Angioplasty and stenting for restenosis after carotid endarterectomy. Initial experience. Stroke 1996;27:2075–2079.

Yusuf S, Sleight P, Pogue J, Bosch J, Davies R, Dagenais G: Effects of an angiotensin-converting-enzyme inhibitor, ramipril, on cardiovascular events in high-risk patients. The Heart Outcome Prevention Evaluation Study Investigators. N Engl J Med 2000;342:145–153.

Yusuf S, Zhao F, Mehta SR, Chrolavicius S, Tognoni G, Fox KK: Clopidogrel in unstable angina to prevent recurrent events trial investigators. N Engl J Med 2001;345:494–502.

Part 3

Cerebrovascular Diseases

Cerebrovasc Dis 2004;17(suppl 2):30–46
DOI: 10.1159/000074818

Acute Treatment of Ischaemic Stroke

Danilo Toni Angel Chamorro Markku Kaste Kennedy Lees
Nils Gunnar Wahlgren Werner Hacke
for the EUSI Executive Committee and the EUSI Writing Committee

Introduction

Despite the proven efficacy of risk factor control and secondary prevention in preventing first-ever or recurrent strokes, stroke incidence in specific age subgroups [Johansson et al., 2000] and stroke hospitalization [Fang and Alderman, 2001] have increased in the last decade. Hence, treatment of acute ischaemic stroke remains essential in order to improve outcome and to lower mortality.

There are 5 main areas in the treatment of acute stroke. The first is the treatment of general conditions that need to be stabilized, which is usually defined as 'general therapy'. The second is specific therapy directed against particular aspects of stroke pathogenesis. Since stroke is mainly caused by acute local or embolic vascular occlusion, one of these aspects is recanalization. Another approach is neuroprotection, which aims to prevent/treat the mechanisms leading to death of neurons in the ischaemic brain. The third main area of stroke treatment is prophylaxis and treatment of complications, which may be either neurological (such as secondary haemorrhage, space-occupying oedema or seizures) or medical (such as aspiration, infections, decubital ulcers or pulmonary embolism). All these aspects of acute stroke treatment will be covered in this article. The fourth area is early secondary prevention to reduce the incidence of early stroke recurrence in the same or another arterial territory. Apart from treatment of increased blood pressure and from the use of anticoagulation, however, early secondary prevention does not substantially differ from secondary prevention in general, for which we refer the reader to the second article of this series. The fifth and final area is early rehabilitation, which has already been covered in the first article of this series of recommendations.

Initial Patient Assessment

When a patient with a focal neurological deficit is first seen, the key questions to be answered are: (1) Is it a stroke? (2) Is there a life-threatening concomitant disease? (3) What kind of stroke is this? (4) Where in the brain is it? (5) What is the pathogenic subtype? (6) What is the prognosis?

The differential diagnosis with non-stroke pathologies always requires CT or MRI. This is also true for the differential diagnosis between ischaemic and haemorrhagic stroke, since the clinical diagnosis of parenchymal haemorrhage is unreliable [Allen 1983; Poungvarin et al., 1991; Weir et al., 1994]. Differentiating a stroke from a transient ischaemic attack (TIA) may be important in the emergency setting, when a decision to give thrombolysis has to be taken. In 60% of TIAs, signs and symptoms completely clear within 1 h of onset, while patients with a deficit persisting for at least 60 min have less than a 2% chance of resolving spontaneously during any subsequent 1-hour period [Levy, 1988]. Moreover, in the NINDS

KARGER
Fax + 41 61 306 12 34
E-Mail karger@karger.ch
www.karger.com

1015–9770/04/0176–0030$21.00/0

Accessible online at:
www.karger.com/ced

trial, among placebo-treated patients who did not completely recover within 1 h or rapidly improve within 3 h, only 2% had complete resolution within 24 h [Marler et al., 2000]. In most TIA patients, no brain tissue damage can be seen with diffusion-weighted (DW) MRI performed when symptoms are still present, while DW lesions are evident in those with longer duration of symptoms, with a lesion visible in follow-up MRI in half of cases [Kidwell et al., 1999].

Clinical examination, with the eventual supplement of neurovascular evaluation of extra- and intracranial vessels, may give some indication on whether the infarct is in the anterior or posterior circulation, while clinical differentiation of ischaemic stroke subtypes is unreliable in the emergency setting [Madden et al., 1995]. In particular, the differentiation between lacunar and non-lacunar (i.e., large artery atherothrombotic or cardioembolic) infarcts based on the clinical syndrome dramatically loses accuracy as the delay in patient neurological examination reduces from days [Bamford et al., 1987, 1991] to a few hours [Toni et al., 1994a, 2000; Toni, 2002] after stroke onset. Patient evaluation with multimodal neuroimaging techniques including DW and perfusion-weighted MRI and MR angiography may significantly improve the differential diagnosis [Ay et al., 1999a, b; Lee et al., 2000; Gerraty et al., 2002].

Clinical examination may quantify the severity of clinical presentation, which is strongly related to late clinical outcome, though less well to early clinical course. In fact, with the exception of patients presenting with stupor or coma who almost always have a bad outcome, usually the severity of neurological deficit a few hours after stroke onset does not allow the differentiation between patients who may deteriorate and those who may improve in the subsequent 48 h [Toni et al., 1995, 1997]. Imaging techniques such as CT [Toni et al., 1995, 1997; Krieger et al., 1999], angiography [Toni et al., 1995], CT perfusion [Wintermark et al., 2000] and particularly DW and perfusion-weighted MRI and MR angiography [Oppenheim et al., 2000; Baird et al., 2001; Arenillas et al., 2002] may be of help in drawing prognostic estimates on which to tailor therapeutic choices in the emergency setting.

However, this variable clinical course, in terms of both clinical picture and clinical severity, may be explained by the dynamic nature of the ischaemic penumbra and by the influence that intracerebral and systemic factors may have on its fate, stressing the key role of the stabilization of patient conditions by general treatment as detailed below.

Monitoring of Vital Neurological Functions in the Stroke Unit or in the Normal Ward

In all stroke patients, neurological status and vital functions (blood pressure, pulse rate, temperature) should be continuously or regularly monitored.

Neurological status is best monitored using validated scales/subscales [Lyden et al., 1994; Lindstrom et al., 1991], which have demonstrated a good correlation with the volume of the underlying infarct [Brott et al., 1989] and with the long-term outcome [Muir et al., 1999; DeGraba et al., 1999; Lindstrom et al., 1991]. An additional value of these scales is that they can also be administered by appropriately trained non-neurologists, if the stroke patient is referred to a normal ward, and by stroke nurses.

The opportunity to submit all stroke patients to instrumental monitoring is largely debated, particularly due to different resource availability in different countries and centres. A reasonable compromise is that online ECG monitoring is advisable in selected cases with past medical history of cardiac disease and/or arrhythmias and in case of haemodynamic instability. The electrodes for cardiac monitoring can also be used for respiratory monitoring, which may be necessary given the frequent episodes of sleep apnoeas or hypopnoeas of acute stroke patients [Iranzo et al., 2002; Turkington et al., 2002]. If cardiac and respiratory instrumental monitoring is not feasible, repeat ECG, clinical checks of respiratory function and blood pressure measurements with automatic inflatable sphygmomanometry should be performed. In most circumstances, conventional non-invasive blood pressure monitoring is adequate. Pulse oximetry is useful for continuous monitoring in stroke units. It provides relevant information on the patient respiratory status. A central catheter and occasionally central venous pressure monitoring is needed for patients with severe stroke treated in specialized wards. Via a central venous catheter, indirect information on intravascular volume, cardiac function and compliance within the venous system can be gained.

General Stroke Treatment

The term 'general treatment' refers to treatment strategies which are not exclusive to stroke treatment. It rather describes what has to be done in order to stabilize every critically ill patient. This not only provides an optimum physiological basis upon which specific therapeutic treatment strategies can be built [Brott et al., 1994; Hacke et al., 1995], but also represents per se a cornerstone of stroke treatment, by treating systemic problems that may significantly influence stroke outcome.

There is consensus that management of general (internal medical) problems is the basis for stroke treatment [WHO Tasks Force on Stroke and Other Cerebrovascular Disorders, 1989; Brott and Reed, 1989; Adams et al., 1994; The European Ad Hoc Consensus Group, 1996]. General management of stroke patients comprises respiratory and cardiac care, fluid and metabolic management, blood pressure control and perhaps treatment of elevated intracranial pressure (ICP). In addition, treatment of seizures and prophylactic measures concerning deep venous thrombosis (DVT), pulmonary embolism, aspiration pneumonia, other infections and decubital ulcer are part of the general treatment of the patients [The European Ad Hoc Consensus Group, 1996, 1997].

Most authors agree that adequate treatment and preservation of vital functions constitute the basis of all therapeutic measures in acute stroke, not only in stroke units, but also in normal wards. On the other hand, one has to keep in mind that even the proposed management of hypertension, hyperglycaemia or fever in stroke patients has never been tested prospectively. It makes sense to keep the patient's general condition in the best physiological shape possible; however, in the past, even this has been controversial, as one can see in the changing attitude towards treatment of elevated blood pressure [Barsan et al., 1989; Adams et al., 1994; Einhäupl et al., 1999].

Pulmonary Function and Airway Protection

Normal respiratory function and adequate blood oxygenation are required for stroke management, since they may be important for the preservation of metabolic function in the ischaemic penumbra. Although there is no convincing prospective clinical evidence that oxygen supply at low flow rates is useful in human brain infarction, [Ronning and Guldvog, 1999], respiratory function has to be monitored in order to detect and treat hypoxia. This may be consequent to extensive vertebrobasilar or hemispheric infarction, large intracranial haemorrhages, sustained seizure activity following hemispheric stroke or complications such as severe pneumonia particularly in patients at risk of aspiration, heart failure, pulmonary embolism or exacerbation of chronic obstructive airway disease. Blood gas analysis or an expiratory pCO_2 and transcutaneous O_2 assessment should be performed early in selected patients with severe stroke and/or impaired pulmonary function. Ventilation may be particularly compromised during sleep, with episodes of sleep apnoeas or hypopnoeas, which may be responsible for early neurological deterioration [Iranzo et al., 2002]. Continuous transdermal pulse oxymetry may provide useful information; however, peripheral oxygen saturation of 90% or higher does not necessarily reflect the situation within the brain, particularly within the deep white matter. Blood oxygenation is improved by the administration of 2–4 litres of O_2/min via a nasal tube and by the use of bronchodilators, when indicated. If there is no pathological respiratory pattern and the blood gas analysis reveals only moderate hypoxaemia, the administration of oxygen is probably sufficient. Non-invasive continuous positive airway pressure via nasal or face mask might be used in case of obstructive sleep apnoea [Iranzo et al., 2002; Turkington et al., 2002], though its actual efficacy should be tested more accurately.

In the event of a pathological respiratory pattern, severe hypoxaemia or hypercarbia, and for the unconscious patient (Glasgow Coma Scale ≤ 8) at high risk for aspiration, early endotracheal intubation may be necessary. Prognosis of stroke patients undergoing intubation is not invariably bad [Grotta et al., 1995; Berrouschot et al., 2000], with some series reporting a 1-year survival rate of about one third of the patients [Steiner et al., 1997]. Of course, before intubation is performed, the general prognosis, co-existing life-threatening medical conditions and the presumed will of the patient and his/her family have to be taken into account.

Cardiac Care and Blood Pressure Management

The existence of a strict heart-brain interaction is well known [Oppenheimer and Hachinsky, 1992a]. Cardiac arrhythmias secondary to stroke, particularly atrial fibrillation [Broderick et al., 1992; Vingerhoets et al., 1993], are not unusual, while sudden death, heart failure and acute myocardial infarction (MI) [Bamford et al., 1990; Broderick et al., 1992] may complicate the clinical course. Significant alterations in the S–T segments and the T waves on the ECG mimicking myocardial ischaemia and Q–T abnormalities may appear in the acute phase [Norris, 1983], and cardiac enzymes may be elevated after stroke [Kaste et al., 1978; James et al., 2000]. In a recent review, it has been reported that while in patients with subarachnoid haemorrhage the ischaemic-like changes and QT prolongation on ECG were mainly a direct consequence of the neurological disease, in patients with ischaemic and haemorrhagic stroke they were more often related to pre-existing coronary artery disease [Khechinashvili and Asplund, 2002]. The routine treatment of this phenomenon, mainly dependent on excess of circulating catecholamines, is β or α/β blocking [Kaste and Roine, in press] when not contraindicated. Finally, irrespective of previous cardiac disease, a correlation has been stressed between infarcts involving the insula and cardiac complications [Oppenheimer et al., 1996].

Every stroke patient should have an initial ECG. Continuous ECG monitoring is advisable in patients with abnormal baseline ECG, past medical history of MI or cardiac arrhythmias, clinical signs/symptoms of myocardial insufficiency and haemodynamic instability.

Subsequently, the intravascular volume must be kept stable. Among the inotropic agents, dobutamine has the advantage of increasing cardiac output without substantially affecting either heart rate or blood pressure. Dopamine may be particularly useful in patients with hypotension or renal insufficiency. Augmentation of cardiac output can increase regional cerebral blood flow (CBF). Increases in cardiac output may increase cerebral perfusion in areas which have lost their autoregulative capacity after acute ischaemia. The use of digitalis is only reasonable when there are obvious signs of myocardial insufficiency. Restoration of normal rhythm by using drugs, cardioversion or pacemaker should be performed, if necessary in co-operation with internists or cardiologists. Optimizing cardiac output with maintenance of a high normal blood pressure and a normal heart rate is the essential basis of stroke management. The central venous pressure should be maintained at approximately 8–10 cm H_2O and its monitoring, although not frequently used in a normal ward, will give early warning of a volume deficiency or volume overload, which both have negative effects on cerebral perfusion.

Blood Pressure Management

Blood pressure monitoring and treatment is likely the most critical issue in general treatment of acute stroke. Contrary to the past attitude in favour of routine blood pressure reduction in every acute stroke patient, at present, blood pressure reduction in the acute setting is handled more cautiously. Data apparently favouring this treatment come from studies suggesting a relationship between high blood pressure and stroke progression [Dávalos et al., 1990], poor functional outcome [Ahmed et al., 2001; Willmot at al., 2002; Leonardi-Bee et al., 2002], increase in brain oedema [Hatashita et al., 1986; Chamorro et al., 1998; Leonardi-Bee et al., 2002] and haemorrhagic transformation of the infarct [Bowes et al., 1996; Fagan et al., 1998]. Moreover, a moderate reduction of blood pressure has been suggested to favour clinical recovery [Chamorro et al., 1998; Scott et al., 2001]. However, evidence contrary to this treatment is also available. Frequently, stroke patients are chronically hypertensive and their brain autoregulatory curve is shifted to the right. This means that while in normal individuals CBF is constant at a mean arterial pressure (MAP) of approximately 80–140 mm Hg, hypertensive stroke patients can better tolerate higher MAP levels, while they are at risk of critical hypoperfusion for MAP levels, usually well-tolerated by normotensive individuals. Furthermore, CBF autoregulation may be defective in an area of evolving infarction [Meyer at al., 1973; Eames et al., 2002] so that flow in the critical penumbra zone is passively dependent on the MAP. Ischaemia/infarction implies a mismatch between blood flow and the metabolic needs of brain tissue. Hence, maintenance of CBF above the infarction threshold is critical in preventing irreversible brain damage. Normal average CBF is approximately 55 ml/100 g/min. Drops in blood pressure must be avoided in order to maintain an adequate cerebral perfusion pressure. This may explain the relationship between low blood pressure at hospital admission and stroke progression [Jorgensen et al., 1994] and bad outcome [Leonardi-Bee et al., 2002], and the correlation between blood pressure decrease induced by nimodipine and bad outcome in the Intravenous Nimodipine West European Stroke Trial [Ahmed et al., 2000]. However, modest reductions in blood pressure with oral perindopril or intravenous sodium nitroprusside or transdermal glyceryl trinitrate apparently did not alter CBF or middle cerebral artery (MCA) flow velocity [Dyker et al., 1997; Butterworth et al., 1998; Rashid et al., 2002].

Finally, elevation of arterial blood pressure may occur in up to 80% of acute stroke patients [Yatsu and Zivin, 1985; Lavin, 1986; Leonardi-Bee et al., 2002], but it is transient and usually spontaneously decreases during the first days [Britton et al., 1986; Jansen et al., 1987; Oppenheimer and Hachinsky, 1992b; Broderick et al., 1993; Harper et al., 1994]. On the other hand, blood pressure increase may be consequent to treatable conditions such as intracranial hypertension, pain, mental stress due to hospitalization and urine retention [Carlberg et al., 1991], and it is sufficient to treat them to obtain an adequate control of blood pressure.

A target systolic blood pressure (SBP) of 180 mm Hg and diastolic blood pressure (DBP) of 100–105 mm Hg is recommended for patients with prior hypertension. In other cases, mild hypertension is desirable (160–180/90–100 mm Hg). Obviously, extremely high blood pressure levels are not acceptable. Systolic values over 220 mm Hg or diastolic values over 120 mm Hg (in some centres, especially in North America, thresholds of 240 mm Hg for SBP and 130 mm Hg for DBP are accepted) constitute an

Table 1. Suggested antihypertensive treatment in acute ischaemic stroke (first 24–48 h), modified from Brott et al. [1994] and Ringleb et al. [1998] (availability of substances may vary between countries)

1	SBP 180–220 mm Hg and/or DBP 105–140 mm Hg	Do not treat
2	SBP ≥220 mm Hg and/or DBP 120–140 mm Hg, on repeated measures	Captopril 6.25–12.5 mg (p.o./i.m.) Labetalol 5–20 mg (i.v.)[1] Urapidil 10–50 mg (i.v.), followed by 4–8 mg/h (i.v.)[2] Clonidine 0.15–0.3 mg (i.v. or s.c.) Dihydralazine 5 mg (i.v.) plus metoprolol 10 mg
3	DBP ≥140 mm Hg	Nitroglycerin 5 mg (i.v.), followed by 1–4 mg/h Sodium nitroprusside 1–2 mg

1 Avoid labetalol in patients with asthma, cardiac failure, severe conduction abnormalities and bradycardia.
2 In patients with unstable conditions and rapidly fluctuating blood pressure, alternating urapidil/arterenol treatment may be used.

indication for early but cautious drug treatment, avoiding a drastic or abrupt reduction of blood pressure.

There are only few indications for immediate antihypertensive therapy. This treatment may be appropriate in the setting of concomitant acute myocardial ischaemia (although extreme lowering of blood pressure is deleterious for MI patients as well), cardiac insufficiency, acute renal failure, acute hypertensive encephalopathy or aortic arch dissection. In patients undergoing thrombolysis or heparin administration, SBP above 180 mm Hg should be avoided. After the CT scan has shown a non-ischaemic cause of stroke, such as subarachnoid haemorrhage, intracerebral haemorrhage or subdural haematoma, antihypertensive treatment may also be started.

Blood pressure values requiring treatment in acute stroke patients and suggested antihypertensive treatments are summarized in tables 1 and 2.

Sublingual calcium antagonists should be avoided because of the risk of abrupt reduction of blood pressure [Grossman et al., 1996], possible ischaemic steal [Ahmed et al., 2000; Adams et al., 1994; Graham, 1982; Power, 1993; Jorgensen et al., 1994] and overshoot hypertension. Oral and intravenous administrations are still frequently used in Europe, although the effects of oral nifedipine are frequently quite substantial, rapid and excessive. The same is true for subcutaneous clonidine. In both cases, the duration of action is hard to predict. Oral captopril (6.25–12.5 mg) has been recommended as an oral first-line drug [Ringleb et al., 1998], but has a short duration of action and can have an abrupt effect. In North America, intravenous labetalol (10 mg), which is available everywhere in Europe, or enalapril are frequently recommended. Excess bradycardia and reduced cardiac output are rare events after labetalol. Intravenous urapidil is increasingly used. Sodium nitroprusside will sometimes become necessary despite some major side-effects, which include reflex tachycardia and coronary artery ischaemia.

For isolated elevation of DBP, nitroglycerine (in Europe) and sodium nitroprusside (in North America) are frequently used, although both are said to increase ICP.

Low or normal-low blood pressure at stroke onset is unusual: it was found only in 5% of patients in the IST trial [Leonardi-Bee et al., 2002]. It may be associated with dehydration, cardiac failure or ischaemia, or sepsis. Blood pressure can be raised by adequate patient rehydration with crystalloid (saline) or, occasionally, colloid solutions. Low cardiac output may need inotropic support.

Glucose Metabolism

An increase in serum glucose levels at hospital admission may be found in 10–20% of patients with normal HbA_{1c} [van Kooten et al., 1993], while 8–20% of stroke patients have a past medical history of diabetes [Toni et al., 1992] and another 5–28% have previously unknown diabetes [Gray et al., 1987]. Hence, hyperglycaemia at stroke onset may be present in 20–50% of cases [Weir et al., 1997].

High glucose levels are harmful in stroke patients [Pulsinelli et al., 1983], having been related to stroke progression [Dávalos et al., 1990], increase in infarct size [Toni et al., 1994b] and poor prognosis [Weir et al., 1997; Capes et al., 2001] independently from stroke severity. This is true not only for diabetic patients, whose metabolic derangement may be dramatically worsened in the acute phase of stroke, but also for non-diabetic subjects. In fact, a recent overview has shown a correlation between even mildly elevated glucose levels of 6.1–7 mmol/l on admission and increased risk of 30-day mortality and poor functional

Table 2. Characteristics of selected antihypertensive drugs that may be used in acute stroke (modified from Kaplan [1990] and Ringleb et al. [1998])

	Dose	Onset, min	Duration, h	Adverse effects
Oral drugs				
Angiotensin-converting enzyme inhibitor				
Captopril	6–12.5 mg sl	15–30	4–6	Decrease in CBF ortostatic hypotension
Parenteral drugs				
Central sympatholytic				
Clonidine	0.2 mg initial then	5–15	6–8	Profound hypotension
	0.1 mg/h up to 0.8 mg (i.v.)			Caution if combined with diuretics
	0.075 mg (s.c.)	5–10	3–5	Initial blood pressure increase, sedation
Vasodilators				
Nitroprusside	0.25–10 μg/kg min^{-1} (i.v.)	1–5		Nausea, vomiting, muscle twitching, sweating, thiocyanate intoxication
Nitroglycerin	5–100 μg/kg min^{-1}	2–5		Tachycardia, headaches, vomiting
Dihydralazin	6.5–20 mg i.v. bolus 1.5–7.5 mg/h i.v. infusion	1–2	1–2	Tachycardia, headaches
β-Blocker				
Propranolol	1–10 mg (i.v.)	1–2	3–6	β-Blocker side-effects (e.g. bronchospasm, decreased cardiac output, bradycardia)
α/β-Blocker				
Labetalol	20–80 mg i.v. bolus 2 mg/min i.v. infusion	5–10	3–5	Vomiting, postural hypotension, nausea, dizziness
α-Blocker				
Urapidil	10–50 mg i.v. bolus 9–30 mg/h i.v. infusion	2–5	3	No serious side-effects

The use of oral calcium antagonists is strongly discouraged.

recovery in non-diabetic patients [Capes et al., 2001]. Hence, temporary insulin treatment may become necessary. A blood glucose level equal to or above 200 mg/dl or 10 mmol/l justifies immediate insulin titration. Unless the blood glucose level is known, no glucose solution should be given to a stroke patient. A pilot study on patients with mild to moderate hyperglycaemia (plasma glucose between 7.0 and 17.0 mmol/l), randomized to receive either a 24-hour infusion of 0.9% (154 mmol/l) saline or a 10% glucose potassium insulin infusion at 100 ml/h, showed that glucose potassium insulin was safe producing a physiological but attenuated glucose response to acute stroke [Scott et al., 1999]. On the other hand, hypoglycaemia can rarely mimic an acute ischaemic infarction [Huff, 2002] and its focal signs are not always those of a seizure. Hence, hypoglycaemia should be treated by an intravenous bolus of dextrose or infusion of 10–20% glucose, preferably via a central venous line.

Body Temperature

Body temperature increases in up to 50% of patients over the initial 48 h of stroke onset [Corbett et al., 2000]. Experimentally, fever increases infarct size [Fukuda et al., 1999], and it is known that high body temperature may favour stroke progression [Castillo et al., 1999] and long-term bad outcome [Reith et al., 1996; Hajat et al., 2000]. In contrast with this observation, it has recently been published that the increase in body temperature is consequent to a severe brain infarct and is not per se responsible for the bad outcome [Boysen and Christensen, 2001]. On the other hand, it is known that hyperthermia, as well as for example hyperglycaemia, is part of the acute phase response, but this does not exclude that it may in turn aggravate stroke prognosis. It has also to be remembered that infection is a risk factor for stroke [Syrjanen et al., 1988; Grau et al., 1995] and that in 60–85% of cases, fever is consequent to an infection after stroke [Grau et al., 1999; Georgilis et al., 1999]. Hence, search of a possible infection (site and nature) is recommended in order to start tailored treatment, while antibiotic, antimycotic or antiviral prophylaxis is not recommended in immunocompetent patients.

Though small randomized studies with high-dose antipyretics provide contradictory data on the usefulness of this approach [Dippel et al., 2001; Kasner et al., 2002], treating an elevated temperature in stroke patients is advisable. Antipyretics such as paracetamol and the early use of antibiotics in cases of apparent bacterial infection such as urinary tract infection or aspiration pneumonia are usually recommended. Although there are no prospective data, one may consider lowering body temperature as soon as it reaches 37.5 °C.

Fluid and Electrolyte Management

Maintaining a balanced fluid and electrolyte status in stroke patients is fundamental to avoid plasma volume contraction, which may influence brain perfusion and kidney function. Moderate or severe dehydration on admission is not uncommon and may be related to bad outcome [Bhalla et al., 2000]. It may be due to pre-existing dehydration, pre-stroke use of diuretics, dysphagia and hyperthermia, the extreme paradigm being those patients found lying on a floor for hours or days. Virtually all acute stroke patients need intravenous fluid therapy, with a more or less positive balance according to the level of dehydration as indicated by haematocrit and osmolality. However, excessive volume replacement may lead to cardiac decompensation and pulmonary oedema in patients with a history of cardiopathy. A slightly negative fluid balance (about 300–500 ml negative balance daily) is usually recommended in the presence of brain oedema with or without evidence of raised intracerebral pressure.

Hypotonic solutions (NaCl 0.45% or glucose 5%) are contraindicated due to the risk of brain oedema increase consequent to reduction of plasma osmolality. Moreover, glucose solutions are not recommended due to the above-mentioned detrimental effects of hyperglycaemia.

Severe electrolyte abnormalities are not frequent in patients with ischaemic stroke [Diringer, 1992]. However, electrolytes should be monitored daily since, although not frequently, hyponatraemia may occur due to the syndrome of inappropriate antidiuretic hormone secretion or to the cerebral salt wasting syndrome [Kaste and Roine, in press]. While the syndrome of inappropriate antidiuretic hormone secretion is managed by fluid restriction or administration of hypertonic saline, the cerebral salt wasting syndrome requires volume and sodium loading. As a rule of thumb, fluid restriction is almost never indicated in acute stroke.

During intravenous insulin administration in order to correct marked hyperglycaemia, concomitant potassium infusion is usually required to prevent hypokalaemia.

Peripheral venous access is usually sufficient for initial fluid management, while a central venous catheter is required in case of infusion of larger volumes of fluids, high osmolality solutions or irritant substances. When high fluid volumes and high concentrations of electrolytes are infused, continuous ECG monitoring must be available.

Recommendations (All Recommendations Are Level IV)

1 Continuous cardiac monitoring is recommended in the first 48 h of stroke onset, particularly in patients with: previous known cardiopathies, history of arrhythmias, unstable blood pressure, clinical signs/symptoms of heart failure, abnormal baseline ECG, and infarct involving the insular cortex.
2 Oxygenation monitoring with pulse oxymetry is recommended.
3 O_2 administration is recommended in case of hypoxaemia (SaO_2 <92% at blood gas analysis or pulse oxymetry).
4 Intubation is recommended in case of potentially reversible respiratory insufficiency.
5 Routine blood pressure lowering is not recommended, except for extremely elevated values (SBP: >200–220 mm Hg or DBP: 120 mm Hg for ischaemic stroke, >180/105 mm Hg for haemorrhagic stroke) confirmed by repeated measurements.
6 Immediate antihypertensive therapy is recommended in case of stroke and heart failure, aortic dissection, acute myocardial infarction, acute renal failure, thrombolysis or intravenous heparin, but should be applied cautiously.
7 Recommended target blood pressure in patients: with prior hypertension: 180/100–105 mm Hg; without prior hypertension: 160–180/90–100 mm Hg, and under thrombolysis: avoid SBP above 180 mm Hg.
8 Recommended drugs for blood pressure treatment: intravenous labetalol or urapidil, intravenous sodium nitroprusside or nitroglycerin, and captopril (p.o.).
9 Avoid nifedipine and any drastic blood pressure decrease.
10 Avoid and treat hypotension, particularly in unstable patients, by administering adequate amounts of fluids and, when required, volume expanders and/or catecholamines (epinephrine 0.1–2 mg/h plus dobutamine 5–50 mg/h).
11 Monitoring of serum glucose levels is recommended, particularly in known diabetic patients.
12 Solutions are not recommended due to the detrimental effects of hyperglycaemia.
13 Treatment of serum glucose levels >10 mmol/l with insulin titration is recommended.
14 Immediate correction of hypoglycaemia is recommended with intravenous dextrose bolus or 10–20% glucose infusion.
15 Treatment of body temperature ≥37.5 °C is recommended.
16 In case of fever, the search of a possible infection (site and aetiology) is recommended in order to start tailored antibiotic treatment.
17 An antibiotic, antimycotic or antiviral prophylaxis is not recommended in immunocompetent patients.
18 Monitoring and correction of electrolyte and fluid disturbances are recommended.
19 Hypotonic solutions (NaCl 0.45% or glucose 5%) are contraindicated due to the risk of brain oedema increase consequent to reduction of plasma osmolality.

None of the recommendations concerning general treatment has been verified in placebo-controlled, randomized, blinded studies. However, the proven efficacy of stroke units to some extent may be consequent to the adherence to guidelines for general treatment, which may be used as an indirect proof of the efficacy of general treatment procedures.

Specific Treatment

Thrombolytic Therapy

Intravenous Recombinant Tissue Plasminogen Activator

Thrombolytic therapy with recombinant tissue plasminogen activator (rt-PA; 0.9 mg/kg body weight) given within 3 h after stroke onset to patients with acute ischaemic stroke significantly improves outcome [The National Institute of Neurological Disorders and Stroke rt-PA Stroke Study Group, 1995], with a number needed to treat of 7.

There have thus far been 17 completed randomized, controlled trials of thrombolytic therapy versus control in 5,216 patients. Of these, 8 trials tested rt-PA in 2,889 patients (56% of all data). Overall, there was an increase in the odds of death with thrombolysis (OR 1.31, 95% CI 1.13–1.52), but this increase was not significant in patients receiving rt-PA. Moreover, despite this, there was a significant reduction in the number of patients with a poor functional outcome (combined death or dependency) at the end of follow-up (OR 0.83, 95% CI 0.73–0.94), which was slightly better in patients receiving rt-PA. Most of the data came from trials testing thrombolysis up to 6 h after stroke, but the subgroup of patients treated within 3 h showed a greater reduction in poor functional outcome with thrombolysis (OR 0.58, 95% CI 0.46–0.74) with no adverse effect on death [Wardlaw and Warlow, 1999; Wardlaw, 2001].

A pooled analysis of individual data of the 4 larger rt-PA trials confirms that thrombolysis works at least up to 4.5 h and potentially up to 6 h after stroke onset [The ATLANTIS, ECASS, and NINDS rt-PA Study Group Investigators, 2003]. Caution is advised before giving intravenous rt-PA to persons with severe stroke (NIH Stroke Scale score >22) or if the CT demonstrates extended early changes of a major infarction, such as sulcal effacement, mass effect and oedema. Early ischaemic changes (EICs) are prevalent within 3 h of stroke onset and correlate with stroke severity. However, EICs are not independently associated with increased risk of adverse outcome after rt-PA treatment, suggesting that EICs on CT scan are not critical to the decision to treat otherwise eligible patients with rt-PA within 3 h of stroke onset [Patel et al., 2001].

Thrombolytic therapy should only be given if the diagnosis is established by a physician who has expertise in the diagnosis of stroke, and a CT of the brain is assessed by physicians who have expertise in reading this imaging study. Because the use of thrombolytic drugs carries the hazard of major bleeding, the risks and potential benefits of rt-PA should be discussed whenever possible with the patient and family before treatment is initiated.

Intravenous administration of rt-PA more than 3 h after stroke should only be given as an experimental therapy following an institutional protocol or within a multicentre clinical trial.

Other Thrombolytic Approaches

Intravenous streptokinase has been shown to be associated with an unacceptable risk of haemorrhage and haemorrhage-associated death [The Multicenter Acute Stroke Trial – Europe Study Group, 1996; Donnan et al., 1995].

Intra-arterial thrombolytic therapy of occlusions of the proximal part of the MCA, using pro-urokinase, has been shown to be significantly associated with better outcome in a randomized trial. This treatment is safe and efficacious in a 6-hour time window, but it requires superselective angiography and is only available in selected centres [Furlan et al., 1999]. Intra-arterial treatment of acute basilar occlusion with urokinase or rt-PA is frequently used in selected centres, but has not been subjected to a randomized trial [Hacke et al., 1988; Brandt et al., 1996].

Recommendations

1 Intravenous rt-PA (0.9 mg/kg, maximum 90 mg), with 10% of the dose given as a bolus followed by an infusion lasting 60 min, is the recommended treatment within 3 h of onset of ischaemic stroke (level I).

2 benefit from the use of intravenous rt-PA for acute ischaemic stroke beyond 3 h after onset of the symptoms is smaller, but present up to 4.5 h (level I).

3 Intravenous rt-PA is not recommended when the time of onset of stroke cannot be ascertained reliably; this includes persons whose strokes are recognized upon awakening (level IV).

4 Intravenous administration of streptokinase is dangerous and not indicated for the management of persons with ischaemic stroke (level I).

5 Data on the efficacy and safety of any other intravenously administered thrombolytic drugs are not available to provide a recommendation.

6 Intra-arterial treatment of acute MCA occlusion in a 6-hour time window using pro-urokinase results in a significantly improved outcome (level II).

7 Acute basilar occlusion may be treated with intra-arterial therapy in selected centres following an institutional protocol as an experimental therapy or within a multicentre clinical trial (level IV).

Table 3. Remaining indications for heparin treatment after stroke

Stroke due to cardiac emboli with high risk of re-embolization (artificial valves, atrial fibrillation, MI with mural thrombi, left atrial thrombosis)
Coagulopathies such as protein C and S deficiency, APC resistance
Symptomatic dissection of extracranial arteries
Symptomatic extra- and intracranial stenoses
Symptomatic internal carotid stenosis prior to operation
Crescendo TIAs or stroke in progression
Sinus venous thrombosis

Defibrinogenating Enzymes

Ancrod, a defibrinogenating enzyme, has been shown to improve outcome after acute ischaemic stroke if given within 3 h after stroke onset and over 5 days [Sherman et al., 2000]. Recently, a European trial testing ancrod treatment in a 6-hour time window has been terminated prematurely not confirming the US findings.

Recommendation

1 Ancrod cannot presently be recommended for use in acute ischaemic stroke outside the setting of clinical trials.

Aspirin

The results of two very large randomized, non-blinded intervention studies indicate that aspirin given within 48 h after stroke (International Stroke Trial, Chinese Acute Stroke Trial) seems to reduce mortality and rate of recurrent stroke minimally, but statistically significantly [International Stroke Trial Collaborative Group, 1997; Chinese Acute Stroke Trial, 1997], with a number needed to treat of 111. Whether the mild positive effect of early aspirin is due to an effect on the infarct itself or due to prevention of recurrent infarction is not yet clear.

Early Anticoagulation

Early anticoagulation with unfractionated heparin (UFH) has been used frequently in treatment after acute ischaemic stroke. However, none of the early anticoagulation trials that had been performed in the past years selected full anticoagulant doses of intravenous UFH as the therapeutic option. Rather, low or moderate doses of subcutaneous UFH were selected and treatment could be delayed for 48 h [International Stroke Trial Collaborative Group, 1997]. Several studies that used intravenous heparinoids [The TOAST Publication Committee, 1998] or subcutaneous low-molecular-weight heparins such as nadroparin [Kay et al., 1995; Hommel et al., 1998], certoparin [Diener et al., 2001], tinzaparin [Bath et al., 2001] or dalteparin [Berge et al., 2000] failed to show a benefit of treatment. While there was some kind of improvement in the outcome or reduction in stroke recurrence rates, this was almost always counterbalanced by an increased number of haemorrhagic complications. Moreover, the higher bleeding rates were obtained in trials that assessed unadjusted low-molecular-weight heparins. In the past 10 years, no randomized studies were performed to test the effects of early full anticoagulation with UFH following acute ischaemic stroke, although such a trial is currently underway [Major Ongoing Stroke Trials, 2002].

In addition, many investigators believe that heparin is not a standard therapy for all stroke subtypes. However, in patients with stroke associated with atrial fibrillation, functional recovery was improved the sooner heparin was administered [Chamorro et al., 1999]. The results obtained in this observational study suggest that in addition to its role to prevent early stroke recurrence, UFH also has therapeutic properties [Chamorro, 2001], including down-regulation of inflammatory markers [Chamorro et al., 2002].

Table 3 gives some indications as to when full-dose intravenous heparin may currently be proposed. While it is recommended to elevate the activated partial thromboplastin time (aPTT) up to twice the individual baseline, it is very important to standardize aPTT ratios to heparin levels, as thromboplastins used to calibrate aPTT values vary significantly among local laboratories. Heparin should only be given as long as it takes to decide on the appropriate secondary prevention. Traditionally, contraindications for the treatment with heparin include large infarcts (e.g. more than 50% of the MCA territory), uncontrollable arterial hypertension and advanced microvascular changes in the brain, although other studies negate these observations and emphasize to maintain aPTT within targeted values for safer use [Chamorro et al., 1995].

Haemodilution

Isovolaemic haemodilution that lowers the haematocrit by 15% or more results in reductions in blood viscosity and improvements in CBF. Several large clinical trials of isovolaemic haemodilution were unable to demonstrate a decline in mortality or disability with treatment [Scandinavian Stroke Study Group, 1987; Italian Acute Stroke Study Group, 1988; The Hemodilution in Stroke Study Group, 1989; Strand, 1992]. Hypervolaemic haemodilution has been examined in small randomized trials with conflicting results. The clinical benefit of haemodilution therapy has not been established, and the possibility of excess brain oedema has not been excluded.

Neuroprotection

No neuroprotective trial has shown improved outcome after stroke on its predefined primary endpoint. A recent pooled analysis of the citicoline trial results suggests some effect on relevant outcome parameters, including MRI data [Dávalos et al., 2002].

Currently, there is no recommendation to treat patients with neuroprotective drugs after ischaemic stroke.

Recommendations

1. There is no recommendation for general use of heparin, low-molecular-weight heparin or heparinoids after ischaemic stroke (level I).
2. Full-dose heparin may be used when there are selected indications such as cardiac sources with high risk of re-embolism, arterial dissection or high-grade arterial stenosis prior to surgery (level IV).
3. Aspirin (100–300 mg per day) may be given within 48 h after ischaemic stroke (level I).
4. Haemodilution therapy is not presently recommended for the management of patients with acute ischaemic stroke (level I).
5. Currently, there is no recommendation to treat stroke patients with neuroprotective substances (level I).

Prevention and Treatment of Complications

Acute stroke predisposes to medical complications [Davenport et al., 1996; Langhorne et al., 2000; Weimar et al., 2002] such as pneumonia, urinary tract infections, malnutrition or volume depletion. Patients may also suffer from DVT and pulmonary embolism. Early supportive care and monitoring of physiological parameters may prevent such complications. This is best done in a dedicated stroke unit with experienced staff and early mobilization. Immobility may lead to infections, contractions and decubital ulcers.

Aspiration and Pneumonia

One of the most important risks in the early phase after stroke is pneumonia. [Davenport et al., 1996; Langhorne et al., 2000], which is still burdened by a high fatality rate. The majority of the pneumonias are caused by aspiration [Horner et al., 1988]. Since aspiration may be detectable by videofluoroscopy in as many as 50% of patients during the initial days after stroke onset, oral feeding should be withheld until the patient has demonstrated both intact swallowing with small amounts of water and intact coughing on command. Aspiration is frequently found, both in patients with reduced consciousness and in those with swallowing disturbances. Dysphagia may present in patients with either anterior or posterior circulation stroke. Swallowing can be tested early and safely with a spoonful of water or a small ice cube. Enteral nutrition should be started if deglutition difficulties are noted. Data at present available suggest a superiority of percutaneous enteral gastrostomy (PEG) vs. nasogastric tube, but are insufficient (too few studies and too few patients) [Bath et al., 2002]. Hence, pending the results of the FOOD trial (www.dcn.ed.ac.uk/food), nasogastric tube feeding is worth considering for short-term enteral feeding, but PEG should be inserted once it is clear that protracted enteral feeding will be required. As a rule of thumb, PEG is indicated when abnormal swallowing is predicted for periods longer than 1 month.

Nasogastric or PEG feeding through avoidance of swallowing may be helpful in the prevention of aspiration pneumonia. They do not completely reduce the risk, however, since reflux of liquid feed can itself promote aspiration [O'Mahony and McIntyre, 1995]. Other reasons for pneumonia include hypostasis, diminished cough and immobilization. Frequent changes of the patient's position in bed and pulmonary physical therapy may prevent this type of pneumonia. When pneumonia is suspected or diagnosed, antibiotic treatment has to be started. Local guidelines on treatment of infections in stroke patients should be developed.

Urinary Tract Infection

Urinary tract infection is the most common medical complication of acute cerebral infarction [Davenport et al., 1996; Langhorne et al., 2000]. It is an incidental finding in as many as 40% of patients dying from stroke [Silver et al., 1984]. Urinary retention is frequent in the early phase after stroke and will require insertion of a urine catheter or suprapubic catheter. Otherwise, incontinent patients should be managed with a condom catheter or 'pad and pants'. Vigilant nursing care is required to prevent perineal irritation and ulceration. Early bladder training is essential. The majority of hospital-acquired urinary tract infections are associated with the use of indwelling catheters [Gerberding, 2002]. In non-stroke patients, suprapubic catheters are considered to carry lower risk of infection [Vandoni et al., 1994], whereas intermittent catheterization has not been shown to reduce the risk. Once urinary infection is diagnosed, appropriate antibiotics should be chosen according to local guidelines.

To avoid bacterial resistance, developing prophylactic antibiotics are best avoided.

Pulmonary Embolism and DVT

Prevention of acute pulmonary embolism [Silver et al., 1984] is of major importance in the care of every patient with stroke. Pulmonary embolism is the cause of death in up to 25% of patients dying following ischaemic cerebral infarction, even in patients who otherwise would have had an excellent recovery from the stroke. Clinically evident pulmonary embolism has been variably estimated to affect 1–16% of patients in prospective trials [Gubitz et al., 2000] and 3–30% in observational studies [Davenport et al., 1996]. The low recent estimates presumably reflect modern clinical practice and admission to a stroke unit. The risk of DVT and pulmonary embolism can be reduced by early hydration and early mobilization. Although graded compression stockings are effective in preventing venous thrombo-embolism in surgical patients, their efficacy after stroke is unproven and is the subject of the CLOTS trial (www.dcn.ed.ac.uk/clots/). They carry little risk, however. Whilst subcutaneous heparin or low-molecular-weight heparin reduce venous thrombo-embolism, their effects are counterbalanced by an increase in haemorrhagic complications [Gubitz et al., 2000]. Prophylaxis with subcutaneous low-dose heparin (5,000 IU twice daily) or low-molecular-weight heparins is reasonable in patients at particularly high risk of DVT or pulmonary embolism. Since chest pain and dyspnoea will occur in 70–80% of those patients with documented pulmonary embolism, nurses and physicians should be attentive to those signs. Examination of lower extremities should be performed daily to detect signs of deep vein thrombosis.

Decubital Ulcer

Frequent turning of immobilized patients is useful for prevention of decubital ulcers. The skin of the incontinent patient must be kept dry. For patients at particularly high risk, an air- or fluid-filled mattress system should be used. If the decubitus does not respond to conservative therapy, antibiotic therapy may be justified for several days, preceding definitive surgical debridement.

Seizures

Partial (focal) or secondary generalized epileptic attacks may occur in the acute phase of ischaemic stroke. Seizures may appear in 2.5–42.8% of cases, while epilepsy varies from 3 to 4% of cases [So et al., 1996; Olsen 2001].

Epilepsy develops in about one third of the patients with early-onset seizures and about one half of those with late-onset seizures [Olsen, 2001]. Standard intravenous and oral antiepileptic drugs can be used. Isolated early seizures do not require chronic treatment. There is no evidence that prophylactic anticonvulsive treatment is beneficial.

Agitation

Agitation and confusion are rarely caused by the stroke [Levine and Finklestein, 1982], but are more frequently a symptom of other complications such as fever, volume depletion or infections. Adequate treatment of the underlying cause must precede any type of sedation or antipsychotic treatment.

Recommendations

1. Low-dose subcutaneous heparin or low-molecular-weight heparins should only be considered for patients at high risk of DVT or pulmonary embolism (level II).
2. The incidence of venous thrombo-embolism may be reduced through early rehydration and mobilization and graded compression stockings (level IV).
3. Infections after stroke should be treated with appropriate antibiotics (level IV).
4. Aspiration pneumonia may not be prevented by nasogastric feeding (level IV).
5. Early mobilization is helpful to prevent numerous complications after stroke including aspiration pneumonia, DVT and decubital ulcers (level IV).
6. Administration of anticonvulsants to prevent recurrent seizures is strongly recommended (level III).
7. Prophylactic administration of anticonvulsants to patients with recent stroke who have not had seizures is not recommended (level IV).

Elevated ICP and Brain Oedema

In younger patients with complete MCA infarction, brain oedema and elevated ICP may be a major complication, leading to herniation [Hacke et al., 1996] within 2–4 days after the onset of symptoms with a mortality of about 80% with standard treatment [Rieke et al., 1995; Hacke et al., 1996; Steiner et al., 2001].

However, in general, brain oedema plays a key role in both early [Toni et al., 1995; Dávalos et al., 1999] and late [Dávalos et al., 1999] ischaemic stroke progression, being responsible not only for impairment of the level of consciousness and brain herniation, but also for impairment of other neurological functions (such as motor strength or speech) [Toni et al., 1995; Dávalos et al., 1999].

Brain oedema may be increased by systemic factors such as fever, hyperglycaemia [Kagansky et al., 2001] and high blood pressure [Hatashita et al., 1986], which further stress the opportunity to monitor and correct these variables.

Medical Therapy

A recent meta-analysis of studies with glycerol shows that in patients with definite or possible ischaemic stroke, glycerol was safe and significantly reduced fatality rate during treatment, but not death/dependence at the end of follow-up [Righetti et al., 2002].

As to mannitol, no beneficial nor harmful effects were reported in a meta-analysis which, however, selected only one small trial as fulfilling the meta-analysis inclusion criteria [Bereczki et al., 2001].

Finally, according to another meta-analysis, corticosteroids neither reduced fatality rate nor improved clinical outcome and given for 2 weeks were unsafe [Qizilbash et al., 2002]. Hence, we do not have substantial clinical evidences favouring pharmacological treatment of brain oedema, though it must be noted that all these compounds were tested in old studies and that larger randomized controlled trials would be warranted. This means that, at present, the use of mannitol or glycerol in patients with acute ischaemic stroke is mainly based on the results of experimental studies or of studies on patients with head trauma.

In case ICP monitoring is available, treatment of brain oedema should be aimed at maintaining cerebral perfusion pressure >70 mm Hg [Unterberg et al., 1997]. ICP monitoring, with intraventricular, intraparenchymatous or epidural catheters, is essential particularly in comatose or sedated patients, where clinical assessment is not feasible. ICP monitoring reduces the need for neuroradiological examinations and allows evaluation of the effectiveness of diverse therapeutic approaches, but is strictly limited to intensive care stroke units.

Irrespective of the type of clinical setting, basic management of elevated ICP following stroke includes head positioning at an elevation of up to 30°, avoidance of noxious stimuli, pain relief, appropriate oxygenation and normalizing body temperature. However, since the head-up position may lead to a decrease in MAP and hence of cerebral perfusion pressure, the head position should be individualized and adjusted according to MAP.

When clinical or neuroimaging signs of space-occupying oedema occur, osmotherapy is the first medical treatment. In many European centres, the drug of choice is 10% intravenous glycerol (4 × 250 ml over 30–60 min), while oral administration (4 × 50 ml) is an alternative choice. In North America, osmotic treatment is started with intravenous mannitol, 25–50 g over 20–30 min every 3–6 h. Replacement fluids should be administered to maintain the calculated serum osmolality in the range of 300–320 mosm/l. As mentioned above, hypotonic and glucose-containing solutions should be avoided as replacement fluids. Dexamethasone and other corticosteroids are not used for brain oedema treatment after stroke.

Small volumes of hypertonic solutions appear to have positive effects on ICP [Shackford et al., 1992; Schwarz et al., 1998, 2002], but this approach would be more efficacious in post-traumatic or post-surgery oedema than in that consequent to ischaemic or haemorrhagic stroke [Qureshi et al., 1998]. Data at present available are insufficient to provide definite indications in patients with neurological damage [Prough and Zornow, 1998].

In intubated patients, short-acting barbiturates such as thiopental given as a bolus can quickly and significantly reduce ICP, by reducing intracranial blood volume, but the effect is short lived and may be exploited only to treat an acute crisis, e.g. prior to operation only. Moreover, barbiturate treatment requires monitoring of ICP and EEG and careful monitoring of haemodynamic parameters, as a significant blood pressure drop may occur. Usually, adrenergic substances must be given to counteract this side-effect. Continuous barbiturates are of no value and may have detrimental long-term effects [Hacke et al., 1995]. Tris-hydroxy-methyl-amino methane buffer solution infused via a central venous catheter and under ICP control may be used after osmotherapy and barbiturate failure. Another approach in case of severely compromised cerebral perfusion pressure could be volume loading by inducing hypertension with vasopressors, but it requires invasive haemodynamic monitoring and intensive care facilities and may be at risk of inducing vasospasm [Kaste and Roine, in press].

Hypothermia

There is experimental evidence that hypothermia is protective after global and focal hypoxic injury to the brain [Busto et al., 1987]. Recently, it has been shown that hypothermia is neuroprotective after cardiac arrest [Bernard et al., 2002; The Hypothermia after Cardiac Arrest Study Group, 2002]. In patients with severe ischaemic stroke in the MCA territory, mild hypothermia (i.e. brain temperature between 32 and 33°C) led to a case fatality rate much lower than expected from natural history of this group of patients. Pneumonia and increase in ICP during rewarming were the only severe side-effects [Schwab et al., 1998]. Similar results have recently been published from a multicentre observational study, which described 50 prospective patients with cerebral infarction involving at least the complete MCA territory treated with moderate hypothermia. Overall mortality rate was 38%: 8% of patients died during hypothermia, due to severe coagulopathy, cardiac failure or uncontrollable intracranial hypertension and 30% died during rewarming due to uncontrollable ICP increase. Neurological outcome of survivors was a mean NIHSS score of 29 and a mean Rankin Scale score of 2.9 (range 2–5) 4 weeks and 3 months after stroke, respectively [Schwab et al., 2001]. Hypothermia affects virtually every organ system. Ventricular ectopy and fibrillation limit the extent of hypothermia, but this is only known to occur at temperatures below 30 °C. The most frequent complications of moderate hypothermia described in the multicentre trial were thrombocytopenia (70%), bradycardia (62%) and pneumonia (48%). The trial does not allow to draw any outcome conclusions, due to the small number of studied patients, but it demonstrates that moderate hypothermia is feasible and worth being tested in multicentre prospective randomized studies.

However, it has recently been reported that after stroke, hypothermia carries a higher risk profile than decompressive surgery [Georgiadis et al., 2002].

Decompressive Surgery

Malignant MCA Infarction

The rationale of decompressive surgery is to allow expansion of the oedematous tissue away from the lateral ventricle, the diencephalon and the mesencephalon in order to reduce ICP, to increase perfusion pressure and to preserve CBF by preventing further compression of the collateral vessels. These factors may help to increase CBF in areas surrounding ischaemic regions, thereby preventing further brain tissue necrosis. In large prospective uncontrolled case series, surgical decompressive therapy in hemispheric space-occupying infarction lowered mortality from roughly 80% down to 40% without increasing the rate of severely disabled survivors [Rieke et al., 1995; Mori 2001]. Early decompressive surgery (e.g. within the first 24 h after stroke onset) can even more markedly reduce case fatality [Schwab et al., 1998]. A prospective, multicentre study protocol has recently been developed and is now underway.

Cerebellar Infarction

Ventriculostomy to reveal hydrocephalus and decompressive surgery is considered the treatment of choice of a space-occupying cerebellar infarction, although the scientific basis for this is by no means any more solid than in hemispheric infarction.

Space-occupying cerebellar infarcts are caused by uni- or bilateral posterior inferior cerebellar artery occlusion or by bilateral superior cerebellar artery occlusion.

Comatose patients with space-occupying cerebellar infarctions have a mortality of about 80% if treated conservatively. This high mortality can be lowered down to 30% if decompressive surgery is performed [Heros, 1992]. Like in space-occupying supra-tentorial infarction, the operation should be performed before signs of herniation are present. The prognosis among survivors is very good, even if they were comatose when the operation was performed. Most of them regain a Barthel Index score of 85 or higher. It should be noted, however, that these are the results of open, small- or medium-sized case series, one of them prospective [Rieke et al., 1993], but mostly retrospective. Data from a controlled, randomized trial are lacking.

Recommendations

1 Osmotherapy is recommended for patients whose condition is deteriorating secondary to increased ICP, including those with herniation syndromes (level IV).
2 Ventriculostomy or surgical decompression and evacuation of large cerebellar infarctions that compress the brain stem is justified (level III).
3 Surgical decompression and evacuation of a large hemispheric infarction can be a life-saving measure and survivors may have a residual neurological deficit that allows an independent life (level III).

References

Adams H, Brott T, Crowell R, Furlan A, Gomez C, Grotta J, Helgason C, et al: Guidelines for the management of patients with acute ischemic stroke. A statement for healthcare professionals from a special writing group of the Stroke Council, American Heart Association. Stroke 1994;25:1901–1914.

Ahmed N, Nasman P, Wahlgren NG: Effect of intravenous nimodipine on blood pressure and outcome after acute stroke. Stroke 2000;31: 1250–1255.

Ahmed N, Wahlgren G: High initial blood pressure after acute stroke is associated with poor functional outcome. J Intern Med 2001;249:467–473.

Allen CMC: Clinical diagnosis of the acute stroke syndrome. Q J Med 1983;208:515–523.

Arenillas JF, Rovira A, Molina CA, Grive E, Montaner J, Alvarez-Sabin J: Prediction of early neurological deterioration using diffusion- and perfusion-weighted imaging in hyperacute middle cerebral artery ischemic stroke. Stroke 2002;33:2197–2205.

Ay H, Buonanno FS, Rordorf G, Schaefer PW, Schwamm LH, Wu O, Gonzalez RG, et al: Normal diffusion-weighted MRI during stroke-like deficits. Neurology 1999;52:1784–1792.

Ay H, Oliveira-Filho J, Buonanno FS, Ezzeddine M, Schaefer PW, Rordorf G, Schwamm LH, et al: Diffusion-weighted imaging identifies a subset of lacunar infarction associated with embolic source. Stroke 1999;30:2644–1650.

Baird AE, Dambrosia J, Janket S, Eichbaum Q, Chaves C, Silver B, Barber PA, et al: A three-item scale for the early prediction of stroke recovery. Lancet 2001;357:2095–2099.

Bamford J, Dennis M, Sandercock P, Burn J, Warlow C: The frequency, causes and timing of death within 30 days of a first stroke. The Oxfordshire Community Stroke Project. J Neurol Neurosurg Psychiatry 1990;53:824–829.

Bamford, J, Sandercock P, Dennis M, Burn J, Warlow C: Classification and natural history of clinically identifiable subtypes of cerebral infarction. Lancet 1991;337:1521–1526.

Bamford J, Sandercock P, Jones L, Warlow CP: The natural history of lacunar infarction: The Oxfordshire Community Stroke Project. Stroke 1987;18:545–551.

Barsan W, Brott T, Olinger C, et al: Early treatment for acute ischemic stroke. Ann Intern Med 1989;111:449–451.

Bath PMW, Bath FJ, Smithard DG: Interventions for dysphagia in acute stroke; in: Cochrane Library, Issue 3, 2002. Update Software.

Bath PM, Lindenstrom E, Boysen G, De Deyn P, Friis P, Leys D, Marttila R, et al: Tinzaparin in acute ischaemic stroke (TAIST): A randomised aspirin-controlled trial. Lancet 2001;358:702–710.

Bereczki D, Liu M, do Prado GF, Fekete I: Mannitol for acute stroke. Cochrane Database Syst Rev 2001;(1):CD001153.

Berge E, Abdelnoor M, Nakstad PH, Sandset PM: Low molecular-weight heparin versus aspirin in patients with acute ischaemic stroke and atrial fibrillation: A double-blind randomised study. HAEST Study Group. Heparin in Acute Embolic Stroke Trial. Lancet 2000;355:1205–1210.

Bernard SA, Gray TW, Buist MD, et al: Treatment of comatose survivors of out-of-hospital cardiac arrest with induced hypothermia N Engl J Med 2002;346:557–563.

Berrouschot J, Rossler A, Koster J, Schneider D: Mechanical ventilation in patients with hemispheric ischemic stroke. Crit Care Med 2000; 28:2956–2961.

Bhalla A, Sankaralingam S, Dundas R, Swaminathan R, Wolfe CD, Rudd AG: Influence of raised plasma osmolality on clinical outcome after acute stroke. Stroke 2000;31:2043–2048.

Boysen G, Christensen H: Stroke severity determines body temperature in acute stroke. Stroke 2001;32:413–417.

Bowes MP, Zivin JA, Thomas GR, Thibodeaux H, Fagan SC: Acute hypertension, but not thrombolysis, increases the incidence and severity of hemorrhagic transformation following experimental stroke in rabbits. Exp Neurol 1996;141: 40–46.

Brandt T, von Kummer R, Müller-Küppers M, Hacke W: Thrombolyic therapy of acute basilar artery occlusion: Variables affecting recanalization and outcome. Stroke 1996;27:875–881.

Britton M, Carlsson A, de Faire U: Blood pressure course in patients with acute stroke and matched controls. Stroke 1986;17:861–864.

Broderick J, Brott T, Barsan W, Clarke Haley E, Levy D, Marler J, Sheppard G, Blum C: Blood pressure during the first minutes of focal cerebral ischemia. Ann Emerg Med 1993;22:1438–1343.

Broderick JP, Phillips SJ, O'Fallon WM, Frye RL, Whisnant JP: Relationship of cardiac disease to stroke occurrence, recurrence, and mortality. Stroke 1992;23:1250–1256.

Brott T, Fieschi C, Hacke W: General therapy of acute ischemic stroke; in Hacke W, Hanley DF, Einhäupl K, Bleck TP (eds): Neurocritical Care. Berlin, Springer, 1994, pp 553–577.

Brott T, Marler JR, Olinger CP, Adams HP Jr, Tomsick T, Barsan WG, Biller J, et al: Measurements of acute cerebral infarction: Lesion size by computed tomography. Stroke 1989;20: 871–875.

Brott T, Reed RL: Intensive care for acute stroke in the community hospital setting. Stroke 1989; 20:694–697.

Busto R, Globus MY, Dietrich WD, et al: Effect of mild hypothermia on ischemia-induced release of neurotransmitters in rat brain. Stroke 1989; 20:904–910.

Butterworth RJ, Cluckie A, Jackson SH, Buxton-Thomas M, Bath PM: Pathophysiological assessment of nitric oxide (given as sodium nitroprusside) in acute ischaemic stroke. Cerebrovasc Dis 1998;8:158–165.

Capes SE, Hunt D, MalmbergK, Pathak P, Gerstein HC: Stress hyperglycemia and prognosis of stroke in nondiabetic and diabetic patients: A systematic overview. Stroke 2001;32:2426–2432.

Carlberg B, Asplund K, Hagg E: Factors influencing admission blood pressure levels in patients with acute stroke. Stroke 1991;22:527–530.

Castillo J, Davalos A, Noya M: Aggravation of acute ischemic stroke by hyperthermia is related to an excitotoxic mechanism. Cerebrovasc Dis 1999;9:22–27.

Chamorro A: Immediate anticoagulation in acute focal brain ischemia revisited: Gathering the evidence. Stroke 2001;32:577–578.

Chamorro A, Cervera A, Castillo J, Davalos A, Aponte JJ, Planas AM: Unfractionated heparin is associated with a lower rise of serum vascular cell adhesion molecule-1 in acute ischemic stroke patients. Neurosci Lett 2002;328:229–232.

Chamorro A, Vila N, Asaco C, Blanc R: Heparin in stroke with atrial fibrillation. Arch Neurol 1999;56:1098–1102.

Chamorro A, Vila N, Ascaso C, Elices E, Schonewille W, Blanc R: Blood pressure and functional recovery in acute ischemic stroke. Stroke 1998;29:1850–1853.

Chamorro A, Vila N, Saiz A, Alday M, Tolosa E: Early anticoagulation after large cerebral embolic infarction: A safety study Neurology 1995;45:861–865.

Chinese Acute Stroke Trial (CAST): Randomised placebo-controlled of early aspirin use in 20,000 patients with acute ischaemic stroke. Lancet 1997;349:1641–1649.

Corbett D, Thornhill J: Temperature modulation (hypothermic and hyperthermic conditions) and its influence on histological and behavioral outcomes following cerebral ischemia. Brain Pathol 2000;10:145–152.

Dávalos A, Castillo J, Alvarez Sabin J, Secades JJ, Mercadal J, Lopez S, Cobo E, et al: Oral citicoline in acute ischemic stroke. An individual patient data pooling analysis of clinical trials. Stroke 2002;33:2850–2857.

Dávalos A, Cendra E, Teruel J, Martinez M, Genis D: Deteriorating ischemic stroke: Risk factors and prognosis. Neurology 1990;40:1865–1869.

Dávalos A, Toni D, Iweins F, Lesaffre E, Bastianello S, Castillo J: Neurological deterioration in acute ischemic stroke: Potential predictors and associated factors in the European cooperative acute stroke study (ECASS) I. Stroke 1999;30: 2631–2636.

Davenport RJ, Dennis MS, Wellwood I, Warlow CP: Complications after acute stroke. Stroke 1996;27:415–420.

DeGraba TJ, Hallenbeck JM, Pettigrew KD, Dutka AJ, Kelly BJ: Progression in acute stroke: Value of the initial NIH stroke scale score on patient stratification in future trials. Stroke 1999;30: 1208–1212.

Diener HC, Ringelstein EB, von Kummer R, Langohr HD, Bewermeyer H, Landgraf H, Hennerici M, et al: Treatment of acute ischemic stroke with the low-molecular-weight heparin certoparin: Results of the TOPAS trial. Therapy of Patients with Acute Stroke (TOPAS) Investigators. Stroke 2001;32:22–29.
Dippel DW, van Breda EJ, van Gemert HM, van der Worp HB, Meijer RJ, Kappelle LJ, Koudstaal PJ: Effect of paracetamol (acetaminophen) on body temperature in acute ischemic stroke: A double-blind, randomized phase II clinical trial. Stroke 2001;32:1607–1612.
Diringer MN: Management of sodium abnormalities in patients with CNS disease. Clin Neuropharmacol 1992;15:427–447.
Donnan G, Davis S, Chambers B, Gates P, Hankey G, McNeil J, Rosen D, et al: Trials of streptokinase in severe acute ischaemic stroke. Lancet 1995;345:578–579.
Dyker AG, Grosset DG, Lees K: Perindopril reduces blood pressure but not cerebral blood flow in patients with recent cerebral ischemic stroke. Stroke 1997;28:580–583.
Eames PJ, Blake MJ, Dawson SL, Panerai RB, Potter JF: Dynamic cerebral autoregulation and beat to beat blood pressure control are impaired in acute ischaemic stroke. J Neurol Neurosurg Psychiatry 2002;72:467–472.
Einhäupl K, Diener C, Hacke W, Hennerici M, Ringelstein B: Behandlung des akuten ischämischen Insults. Dtsch Ärztebl 1999;17:1123–1130.
Fagan SC, Bowes MP, Lyden PD, Zivin JA: Acute hypertension promotes hemorrhagic transformation in a rabbit embolic stroke model: Effect of labetalol. Exp Neurol 1998;150:153–158.
Fang J, Alderman MH: Trend of stroke hospitalization, United States, 1988–1997. Stroke 2001; 32:2221–2226.
Fukuda H, Kitani M, Takahashi K: Body temperature correlates with functional outcome and the lesion size of cerebral infarction. Acta Neurol Scand 1999;100:385–390.
Furlan A, Higashida R, Wechsler L, Gent M, Rowley H, Kase C, Pessin M, Ahuja A, Callahan F, Clark WM, Silver F, Rivera F: Intra-arterial prourokinase for acute ischemic stroke. The PROACT II Study: A randomized controlled trial. Prolyse in Acute Cerebral Thromboembolism. JAMA 1999;282:2003–2011.
Georgiadis D, Schwarz S, Aschoff A, Schwab S: Hemicraniectomy and moderate hypothermia in patients with severe ischemic stroke Stroke 2002;33:1584–1588.
Georgilis K, Plomaritoglou A, Dafni U, Bassiakos Y, Vemmos K: Aetiology of fever in patients with acute stroke. J Intern Med 1999;246:203–209.
Gerberding JL: Hospital-onset infections: A patient safety issue. Ann Int Med 2002;137:665–667.
Gerraty RP, Parsons MW, Barber PA, Darby DG, Desmond PM, Tress BM, Davis SM: Examining the lacunar hypothesis with diffusion and perfusion magnetic resonance imaging. Stroke 2002;33:2019–2024.
Graham DI: Ischemic brain damage following emergency blood pressure lowering in hypertensive patients. Acta Med Scand 1982; 678(suppl):61–69.
Grau A, Buggle F, Heindl S, Streichen-Wiehn C, Banerjee T, Maiwald M, Rohlfs M, et al: Recent infection as a risk factor for cerebrovascular ischemia. Stroke 1995;26:373–379.
Grau AJ, Buggle F, Schnitzler P, Spiel M, Lichy C, Hacke W: Fever and infection early after ischemic stroke. J Neurol Sci 1999;171:115–120.
Gray CS, Taylor R, French JM, Alberti KG, Venables GS, James OF, Shaw DA, Cartlidge NE, Bates D: The prognostic value of stress hyperglycaemia and previously unrecognized diabetes in acute stroke. Diabet Med 1987;4:237–240.
Grossman E, Messerli FH, Grodzicki T, Kowey P: Should a moratorium be placed on sublingual nifedipine capsules given for hypertensive emergencies and pseudoemergencies? JAMA 1996;276:1328–1331.
Grotta J, Pasteur W, Khwaja G, Hamel T, Hamel T, Fisher M, Ramirez A: Elective intubation for neurologic deterioration after stroke. Neurology 1995;45:640–644.
Gubitz G, Counsell C, Sandercock P, Signorini D: Anticoagulants for acute ischaemic stroke; in: Cochrane Library, Issue 3, 2000. Update Software.
Hacke W, Schwab S, Horn M, Spranger M, De-Georgia M, von Kummer R: Malignant middle cerebral artery territory infarction: Clinical course and prognostic signs. Arch Neurol 1996; 53:309–315.
Hacke W, Stingele R, Steiner T, Schuchardt V, Schwab S: Critical care of acute ischemic stroke. Intensive Care Med 1995;21:856–862.
Hacke W, Zeumer H, Ferbert A, Brückmann H, Del Zoppo G: Intra-arterial thrombolytic therapy improves outcome in patients with acute vertebrobasilar occlusive disease. Stroke 1988; 19:1216–1222.
Hajat C, Hajat S, Sharma P: Effects of poststroke pyrexia on stroke outcome: A meta-analysis of studies in patients. Stroke 2000;31:410–414.
Harper G, Castleden CM, Potter JF: Factors affecting changes in blood pressure after acute stroke. Stroke 1994;25:1726–1729.
Hatashita S, Hoff JT, Ishii S: Focal brain edema associated with acute arterial hypertension. J Neurosurg 1986;64:643–649.
Heros RC: Surgical treatment of cerebellar infarction. Stroke 1992;23:937–938.
Hommel M, for the FISS bis Investigators group: Fraxiparin in acute ischaemic stroke. Cerebrovasc Dis 1998;8:63–68.
Horner J, Massey E, Riski J, et al: Aspiration following stroke: Clinical correlates and outcome. Neurology 1988;38:1359–1362.
Huff JS: Stroke mimics and chameleons. Emerg Med Clin North Am 2002;20:583–595.
International Stroke Trial Collaborative Group: The International Stroke Trial (IST): A randomised trial of aspirin, subcutaneous heparin, both, or neither among 19,435 patients with acute ischaemic stroke. Lancet 1997;349: 1569–1581.
Iranzo A, Santamaría J, Berenguer J, Sánchez M, Chamorro A: Prevalence and clinical importance of sleep apnea in the first night after cerebral infarction. Neurology 2002;58:911–916.
Italian Acute Stroke Study Group: Haemodilution in acute stroke: Results of the Italian Haemodilution Trial. Lancet 1988;i:318–321.
James P, Ellis CJ, Whitlock RML, McNeil AR, Henley J, Anderson NE: Relation between troponin T concentration and mortality in patients presenting with an acute stroke: Observational study. BMJ 2000;320:1502–1504.
Jansen PAF, Schulte BPM, Poels EFJ, Gribnau FWJ: Course of blood pressure after cerebral infarction and transient ischemic attack. Clin Neurol Neurosurg 1987;89:243–246.
Johansson B, Norrving B, Lindgren A: Increased stroke incidence in Lund-Orup, Sweden, between 1983 to 1985 and 1993 to 1995. Stroke 2000;31:481–486.
Jørgensen HS, Nakayama H, Raaschou HO, Olsen TS: Effect of blood pressure and diabetes on stroke in progression. Lancet 1994;344:156–159
Kagansky N, Levy S, Knobler H: The role of hyperglycemia in acute stroke. Arch Neurol 2001;58: 1209–1212.
Kasner SE, Wein T, Piriyawat P, Villar-Cordova CE, Chalela JA, Krieger DW, Morgenstern LB, et al: Acetaminophen for altering body temperature in acute stroke: A randomized clinical trial. Stroke 2002;33:130–134.
Kaste M, Roine RO: General stroke management and stroke units; in Grotta JC, Choi D, Mohr JP, Weir B, Wolf P (eds): Stroke, Pathophysiology, Diagnosis and Management. Philadelphia, Harcourt Health Sciences, in press.
Kaste M, Somer H, Konttinen A: Heart type creatine kinase isoenzyme (CK MB) in acute cerebral disorders. Br Heart J 1978;40:802–805.
Kay R, Wong KS, Yu YL: Low-molecular-weight heparin for the treatment of acute ischaemic stroke. N Engl J Med 1995;333:1588–1593.
Khechinashvili G, Asplund K: Electrocardiographic changes in patients with acute stroke: A systematic review. Cerebrovasc Dis 2002;14:67–76.
Kidwell CS, Alger JR, Di Salle F, Starkman S, Villablanca P, Bentson J, Saver JL: Diffusion MRI in patients with transient ischemic attacks. Stroke 1999;30:1174–1180.
van Kooten F, Hoogerbrugge N, Naarding P, Koudstaal PJ: Hyperglycemia in the acute phase of stroke is not caused by stress. Stroke 1993;24:1129–1132.
Krieger DW, Demchuk AM, Kasner SE, Jauss M, Hantson L: Early clinical and radiological predictors of fatal brain swelling in ischemic stroke. Stroke 1999;30:287–292.
Langhorne P, Stott DJ, Robertson L, MacDonald J, Jones L, McAlpine C, Dick F, et al: Medical complications after stroke: A multicenter study. Stroke 2000;31:1223–1229.
Lavin P: Management of hypertension in patients with acute stroke. Arch Intern Med 1986;146: 66–68.

Lee LJ, Kidwell CS, Alger J, Starkman S, Saver JL: Impact on stroke subtype diagnosis of early diffusion-weighted magnetic resonance imaging and magnetic resonance angiography. Stroke 2000;31:1081–1089.

Leonardi-Bee J, Bath PMW, Philips SJ, Sandercock PAG, for the IST Collaborative Group: Blood pressure and clinical outcomes in the International Stroke Trial. Stroke 2002;33: 1315–1320

Levine DN, Finklestein S: Delayed psychosis after right temporoparietal stroke or trauma: Relation to epilepsy. Neurology 1982;32:267–273.

Levy DE: How transient are transient ischemic attacks? Neurology 1988;38:674–677.

Lindstrom E, Boysen G, Christiansen LW, Nansen BR, Nielsen PW: Reliability of Scandinavian neurological stroke scale. Cerebrovasc Dis 1991;1:103–107.

Lyden P, Brott T, Tilley B, Welch KM, Mascha EJ, Levine S, Haley EC, et al: Improved reliability of the NIH Stroke Scale using video training. NINDS TPA Stroke Study Group. Stroke 1994;25:2220–2226.

Madden KP, Karanjia PN, Adams, HP Jr, Clarke WR, the TOAST Investigators: Accuracy of initial stroke subtype diagnosis in the TOAST study. Neurology 1995;45:1975–1979.

Major ongoing stroke trials. Stroke 2002;33:646–655.

Major ongoing stroke trials. Stroke 2002;33:2525–2535.

Marler JR, Tilley BC, Lu M, Brott TG, Lyden PC, Grotta JC, Broderick JP, et al: Early stroke treatment associated with better outcome: The NINDS rt-PA stroke study. Neurology 2000; 55:1649–1655.

Meyer JS, Shimazu K, Fukuhuchi, Ohuchi T, Okamoto S, Koto A: Impaired neurogenic cerebrovascular control and dysautoregulation after stroke. Stroke 1973;4:169–173.

Mori K, Aoki A, Yamamoto T, Maeda M: Aggressive decompressive surgery in patients with massive hemispheric embolic cerebral infarction associated with severe brain swelling. Acta Neurochir (Wien) 2001;143:483–492.

Muir KW, Weir CJ, Alwan W, Squire IB, Lees KR: C-reactive protein and outcome after ischemic stroke. Stroke 1999;30:981–985.

Norris J: Effects of cerebrovascular lesions on the heart. Neurol Clin 1983;1:87–101.

O'Mahony D, McIntyre AS: Artificial feeding for elderly patients after stroke. Age Ageing 1995; 24:533–535.

Olsen TS: Post-stroke epilepsy. Curr Atheroscler Rep 2001;3:340–344.

Oppenheimer S, Hachinski V: Complications of acute stroke. Lancet 1992a;339:721–724.

Oppenheimer SM, Hachinsky VC: The cardiac consequences of stroke. Neurol Clin 1992b;10: 167–176.

Oppenheimer SM, Keden G, Martin WM: Left-insular cortex lesions perturb cardiac autonomic tone in humans. Clin Auton Res 1996;6: 131–140.

Oppenheim C, Samson Y, Manai R, Lalam T, Vandamme X, Crozier S, Srour A, et al: Prediction of malignant middle cerebral artery infarction by diffusion-weighted imaging. Stroke 2000; 31:2175–2181.

Patel SC, Levine SR, Tilley BC, Grotta JC, Lu M, Frankel M, Haley EC Jr, et al: National Institute of Neurological Disorders and Stroke rt-PA Stroke Study Group. Lack of clinical significance of early ischemic changes on computed tomography in acute stroke. JAMA 2001;286: 2830–2838.

Poungvarin N, Viriyavejakul A, Komontri C: Siriraj stroke score and validation study to distinguish supratentorial intracerebral haemorrhage from infarction. BMJ 1991;302:1565–1567.

Power WJ: Acute hypertension after stroke: The scientific basis for treatment decisions. Neurology 1993;43:461–467.

Prough DS, Zornow MH: Hypertonic maintenance fluids for patients with cerebral edema: Does the evidence support a 'phase II' trial? Crit Care Med 1998;26:421–422.

Pulsinelli W, Levy D, Sigsbee B, Scherer P, Plum F: Increased damage after ischemic stroke in patients with hyperglycemia with or without established diabetes mellitus. Am J Med 74:540–544.

Qizilbash N, Lewington SL, Lopez-Arrieta JM: Corticosteroids for acute ischaemic stroke. Cochrane Database Syst Rev 2002;(2): CD000064.

Qureshi AI, Suarez JI, Bhardwaj A, Mirski M, Schnitzer MS, Hanley DF, Ulatowski JA: Use of hypertonic (3%) saline/acetate infusion in the treatment of cerebral edema: Effect on intracranial pressure and lateral displacement of the brain. Crit Care Med 1998;26:440–446.

Rashid P, Leonardi-Bee JA, Weaver CS, Bath FJ, Bath PMW: The effect of transdermal glyceryl trinitrate, a nitric oxide donor, on blood pressure and middle cerebral artery blood velocity in acute stroke. Stroke 2002;33:383.

Reith J, Jørgensen H, Pedersen P, Nakayama H, Raaschou H, Jeppesen L, Olsen T: Body temperature in acute stroke: Relation to stroke severity, infarct size, mortality and outcome. Lancet 1996;347:422–425.

Rieke K, Schwab S, Krieger D, von Kummer R, Aschoff A, Schuchardt V, Hacke W: Decompressive surgery in space-occupying hemispheric infarction: Results of an open, prospective trial. Crit Care Med 1995;23:1576–1587.

Righetti E, Celani MG, Cantisani TA, Sterzi R, Boysen G, Ricci S: Glycerol for acute stroke: A Cochrane systematic review. J Neurol 2002; 249:445–451.

Ringleb PA, Bertram M, Keller E, Hacke W: Hypertension in patients with cerebrovascular accident. To treat or not to treat? Nephrol Dial Transplant 1998;13:2179–2181.

Ronning OM, Guldvog B: Should stroke victims routinely receive supplemental oxygen? A quasi-randomized controlled trial. Stroke 1999;30: 2033–2037.

Scandinavian Stroke Study Group: Multicenter trial of hemodilution in acute ischemic stroke. 1. Results in the total patient population. Stroke 1987;18:691–699.

Schwab S, Georgiadis D, Berrouschot J, Schellinger PD, Graffangino C, Mayer SA: Feasibility and safety of moderate hypothermia after massive hemispheric infarction. Stroke 2001;32:2033–2035.

Schwab S, Schwarz S, Spranger M, Keller E, Bertram M, Hacke W: Moderate hypothermia in the treatment of patients with severe middle cerebral artery infarction. Stroke 1998;29: 2461–2466.

Schwarz S, Georgiadis D, Aschoff A, Schwab S: Effects of hypertonic (10%) saline in patients with raised intracranial pressure after stroke. Stroke 2002;33:136–140.

Schwarz S, Schwab S, Bertram M, Aschoff A, Hacke W: Effects of hypertonic saline hydroxyethyl starch solution and mannitol in patients with increased intracranial pressure after stroke. Stroke 1998;29:1550–1555.

Scott JF, Robinson GM, French JM, O'Connell JE, Alberti KG, Gray C: Glucose potassium insulin infusions in the treatment of acute stroke patients with mild to moderate hyperglycemia: The Glucose Insulin in Stroke Trial (GIST). Stroke 1999;30:793–799.

Scott JF, Robinson GM, French JM, O'Connell JE, Alberti KG, Gray CS: Blood pressure response to glucose potassium insulin therapy in patients with acute stroke with mild to moderate hyperglycaemia. J Neurol Neurosurg Psychiatry 2001;70:401–404.

Shackford SR, Zhuang J, Schmoker J: Intravenous fluid tonicity: Effect on intracranial pressure, cerebral blood flow, and cerebral oxygen delivery in focal brain injury J Neurosurg 1992;76: 91–98.

Sherman DG, Atkinson RP, Chippendale T, Levin KA, Ng K, Futrell N, Hsu CY, Levy DE: Intravenous ancrod for treatment of acute ischemic stroke: The STAT study: A randomized controlled trial. Stroke Treatment with Ancrod Trial. JAMA 2000;283:2395–2403.

Silver F, Norris J, Lewis A, Hachinski V: Early mortality following stroke: A prospective review. Stroke 1984;15:492–496.

So EL, Annegers JF, Hauser WA, O'Brien PC, Whisnant JP: Population-based study of seizure disorders after cerebral infarction. Neurology 1996;46:350–355.

Steiner T, Mendoza G, De Georgia M, Schellinger P, Holle R, Hacke W: Prognosis of stroke patients requiring mechanical ventilation in a neurological critical care unit. Stroke 1997;28: 711–715.

Steiner T, Ringleb P, Hacke W: Treatment options for large hemispheric stroke. Neurology 2001; 57:S61–S68.

Strand T: Evaluation of long-term outcome and safety after hemodilution therapy in acute ischemic stroke. Stroke 1992;23:657–662.

Syrjanen J, Valtonen VV, Iivanainen M, Kaste M, Huttunen JK: Preceding infection as an important risk factor for ischaemic brain infarction in young and middle-aged patients. Br Med J (Clin Res Ed) 1988;296:1156–1160.

The ATLANTIS, ECASS, and NINDS rt-PA Study Group Investigators: Better outcome with early stroke treatment: A pooled analysis of ATLANTIS, ECASS, and NINDS rt-PA stroke trials. Lancet 2003; in revision.

The European Ad Hoc Consensus Group: European strategies for early intervention in stroke. Cerebrovasc Dis 1996;6:315–324.

The European Ad Hoc Consensus Group: Optimizing intensive care in stroke: A European perspective. A report of an Ad Hoc Consensus Group meeting. Cerebrovasc Dis 1997;7:113–128.

The Hemodilution in Stroke Study Group: Hypervolemic hemodilution treatment of acute stroke: Results of a randomized multicenter trial using pentastarch. Stroke 1989;20:317–323.

The Hypothermia after Cardiac Arrest Study Group: Mild therapeutic hypothermia to improve the neurologic outcome after cardiac arrest N Engl J Med 2002;346:549–556.

The Multicenter Acute Stroke Trial – Europe Study Group: Thrombolytic therapy with streptokinase in acute ischaemic stroke. N Engl Med 1996;335:145–150.

The National Institute of Neurological Disorders and Stroke rt-PA Stroke Study Group: Tissue plasminogen activator for acute ischemic stroke. N Engl J Med 1995;333:1581–1587.

The TOAST Publication Committee: Low-molecular-weight heparinoid, ORG 10172 and outcome after acute ischemic stroke. JAMA 1998; 279:1265–1272.

Toni D: Hyperacute Diagnosis of subcortical infarction; in Donnan G, Norrving B, Bamford J, Bogousslavsky J (eds): Lacunar and Other Subcortical Infarctions. Oxford University Press, 2002, pp 184–194.

Toni D, Del Duca R, Fiorelli M, Sacchetti ML, Bastianello S, Giubilei F, Martinazzo C, Argentino C: Pure motor hemiparesis and sensorimotor stroke: Accuracy of the very early clinical diagnosis of lacunar strokes. Stroke 1994a;25:92–96.

Toni D, De Michele M, Fiorelli M, Bastianello S, Camerlingo M, Sacchetti ML, Argentino C, Fieschi C: Influence of hyperglycaemia on infarct size and clinical outcome of acute ischemic stroke patients with intracranial arterial occlusion. J Neurol Sci 1994b;123:129–133.

Toni D, Fiorelli M, Bastianello S, Falcou A, Sette G, Ceschin V, Sacchetti ML, Argentino C: Acute ischemic strokes improving during the first 48 hours of onset: Predictability, outcome, and possible mechanisms. A comparison with early deteriorating strokes. Stroke 1997;28:10–14.

Toni D, Fiorelli M, Gentile M, Bastianello S, Sacchetti ML, Argentino C, Pozzilli C, Fieschi C: Progressing neurological deficit secondary to acute ischemic stroke. A study on predictability, pathogenesis, and prognosis. Arch Neurol 1995;52:670–675.

Toni D, Iweins F, von Kummer R, Busse O, Bogousslavsky J, Falcou A, Lesaffre E, Lenzi GL, for the ECASS I Group: Identification of lacunar infarcts before thrombolysis in the ECASS I study. Neurology 2000;54;684–688.

Toni D, Sacchetti ML, Argentino C, Gentile M, Cavalletti C, Frontoni M, Fieschi C: Does hyperglycaemia play a role on the outcome of acute ischaemic stroke patients? J Neurol 1992; 239:382–386.

Turkington PM, Bamford J, Wanklyn P, Elliott MW: Prevalence and predictors of upper airway obstruction in the first 24 hours after acute stroke. Stroke 2002;33:2037–2042.

Unterberg AW, Kiening KL, Hartl R, Bardt T, Sarrafzadeh AS, Lanksch WR: Multimodal monitoring in patients with head injury: evaluation of the effects of treatment on cerebral oxygenation. J Trauma 1997;42:532–537.

Vandoni RE, Lironi A, Tschantz P: Bacteriuria during urinary tract catheterization: Suprapubic versus urethral route: A prospective randomized trial. Acta Chir Belg 1994;94:12–16.

Vingerhoets F, Bogousslavsky J, Regli F, Van Melle G: Atrial fibrillation after acute stroke. Stroke 1993;24:26–30.

Wardlaw JM: Overview of Cochrane thrombolysis meta-analysis Neurology 2001;57(suppl 2): S69–S76.

Wardlaw J, Warlow C: Thrombolytic therapy for acute ischaemic stroke – The updated Cochrane database of systemic reviews metaanalysis. Cerebrovasc Dis 1999;9:124.

Weimar C, Roth MP, Zillessen G, Glahn J, Wimmer ML, Busse O, Haberl RL, Diener HC, German Stroke Date Bank Collaborators: Complications following acute ischemic stroke. Eur Neurol 2002;48:133–140.

Weir CJ, Murray GD, Adams FG, Muir KW, Grosset DG, Lees KR: Poor accuracy of stroke scoring systems for differential clinical diagnosis of intracranial haemorrhage and infarction. Lancet 1994;344:999–1002.

Weir CJ, Murray GD, Dyker AG, Lees KR: Is hyperglycaemia an independent predictor of poor outcome after acute stroke? Results of a long-term follow up study. BMJ 1997;314: 1303–1306.

WHO Task Force on Stroke and Other Cerebrovascular Disorders: Recommendations on stroke prevention, diagnosis, and therapy. Report of the WHO Task Force on Stroke and Other Cerebrovascular Disorders. Stroke 1989;20: 1407–1431.

Willmot M, Leonardi-Bee J, Bath PMW: High blood pressure in acute stroke and subsequent outcome: A systematic review. Cerebovasc Dis 2002;13(suppl 3):95.

Wintermark M, Reichhart M, Thiran J-P, Maeder P, Chalaron M, Schnyder P, Bogousslavsky J, Meuli R: Prognostic accuracy of cerebral blood flow measurement by perfusion computed tomography, at the time of emergency room admission, in acute stroke patients Ann Neurol 2002;51;417–432.

Yatsu FM, Zivin J: Hypertension in acute ischemic strokes. Not to treat Arch Neurol 1985;42:999–1000.